Learn Medical Spanish for Healthcare Professionals

3 Books in 1

Speak Medical Spanish in 30 Days!

THIS COLLECTION INCLUDES THE FOLLOWING BOOKS:

Introduction to Medical Spanish and Basics
Complete Guide To Learn Medical
Spanish in 30 Days!

Spanish Medical Communication:
Terminology, Anatomy, Procedures, Prescription,
and Emergencies

Cultural Competence in Healthcare
and Additional Practice
Building Bridges of Understanding: Cultivating
Cultural Competence in Healthcare and Beyond!

Table of Contents

$100+ FREE BONUSES

**Medical Spanish
Course**

**100 Flashcards
+ 30-Day Study Plan**

**100 Medical Spanish
Audio Pronunciations**

**Real-life Medical
Scenarios**

Scan QR code to claim
your bonuses

—— OR ——

visit bit.ly/3K4VMUt

BOOK

01

Introduction to Medical Spanish and Basics

Complete Guide To Learn Medical
Spanish in 30 Days!

Book 1 Description

Welcome to Introduction to Medical Spanish and Basics, the first part of our groundbreaking series. As a healthcare professional, you hold the key to bridging the communication gap with your Spanish-speaking patients, and this book is your gateway to success!

In 'Introduction', we emphasize the importance of medical Spanish for your career, breaking down barriers and fostering deeper connections with patients. Discover the benefits of bilingualism in healthcare, which opens a world of opportunities in the healthcare landscape.

Join us on an empowering journey to:

- Understand the significance of medical Spanish for healthcare professionals.
- Embrace the advantages of bilingualism in healthcare.
- Explore the book's well-structured content and learning path.
- Follow guidelines for mastering medical Spanish in just 30 days.
- Utilize a suggested study plan tailored to your busy schedule.

Build strong foundations with 'Spanish Basics':

- Master the Spanish alphabet, sounds, vowel sounds, and consonant sounds.
- Learn medical Spanish for greetings, introductions, and essential phrases.
- Acquire effective strategies to confidently retain and use Spanish.
- Practice with exercises and measure progress with the answer key.

Embark on a transformative journey today, unlocking the power of communication in healthcare! This experience will elevate your patient interactions, enrich your professional life, and make a lasting impact on those you serve. Together, let's build a bridge of compassion and inclusivity in healthcare.

Chapter 1:
Introduction

Las palabras abren puertas sobre el mar.

Rafael Alberti

The importance of healthcare professionals learning medical Spanish

Did you know Spanish has become the second most-spoken non-English language in the United States? If this pattern continues, it is anticipated that by 2050, the United States will have surpassed all other nations and will have become the largest Spanish-speaking nation. Additionally, it is anticipated that the Hispanic population will reach 111 million by 2060 (Figure 1), and more than 25 million people in the United States have a limited ability to communicate in English. Mexicans make up the largest Hispanic group in the US, with over 37 million people, followed by Puerto Ricans, Salvadorans, and Cubans. Notably, Venezuelans are the fastest-growing population, with an increase of 169% between 2010 and 2021. This data highlights the diverse backgrounds of the Hispanic population in the U.S., underscoring the need for healthcare providers to be aware of these demographics (Figure 2). Learning Spanish is now necessary for people in many professions, including those who work in fields such as medicine and commerce, as well as those whose primary language is not Spanish. Join the millions of people who are already broadening their linguistic horizons and discover a whole new universe of opportunities by learning a new language.

It is possible that the difficulty of expressing essential medical information with a patient who does not speak your language will become overwhelming for you when you are engaged in hospital activities. Unfortunately, language problems can frequently get in the way of efficient communication, which can then result in misunderstandings, incorrect diagnoses, and insufficient treatment. In addition, clear communication with Spanish-speaking patients is crucial in reducing errors and preventing medical malpractice lawsuits.

It is crucial for medical professionals to communicate clearly and effectively with their patients to ensure they receive the highest possible level of care. Medical personnel can provide higher quality care, boost patient satisfaction, and advance their careers if they can communicate effectively in the patient's native language. However, learning a new language can be time-consuming, and it is not feasible to become fluent in every language that your patients speak. What if you could quickly and easily learn the Spanish words and phrases that are most commonly used in medical situations?

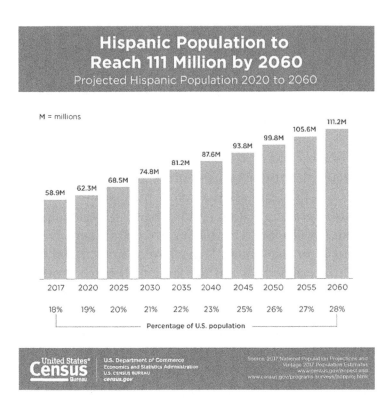

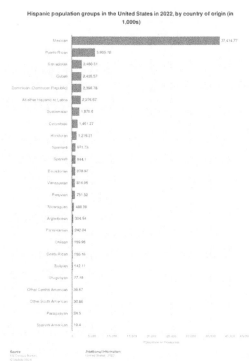

The benefits of being bilingual in healthcare

Bilingual healthcare professionals can serve as cultural intermediaries, facilitating communication between patients and their healthcare providers. Moreover, the acquiring a new language can expand an individual's personal and occupational outlooks, imparting a more profound understanding of diverse cultures and viewpoints.

As previously mentioned, the escalating linguistic heterogeneity within the United States carries extensive ramifications for the healthcare sector. Various remedies have been suggested to tackle this predicament, such as interpreter services, which may incur a substantial expense for medical facilities.

An alternative method involves the utilization of translation aids, such as MediBabble or Google Translate. Nevertheless, these instruments are not infallible and may still generate translation inaccuracies, thereby potentially jeopardizing patients. Additionally, despite the substantial presence of Spanish-speaking individuals in the United States, only a modest percentage of physicians identify as Spanish speakers. This highlights the urgent need for bilingual nursing staff and healthcare interpreters, who can facilitate clear and effective communication of health-related information.

Many healthcare facilities are actively seeking to hire bilingual healthcare professionals, particularly nurses, for many reasons, especially as frontline personnel.

Improving the Quality of Care: Communication fluency is essential to delivering high-quality care in healthcare settings. Speaking in a patient's first or native language can provide many benefits, including:

1. Increasing comfort with the healthcare provider

2. Reducing fears and anxieties related to navigating healthcare settings

3. Receiving critical medical information in one's native language

4. Asking questions in one's native language

5. Advocating for one's needs in the full expression of one's native language

6. Demonstrating respect and cultural competency

Cultural competency is vital to respecting, understanding, and effectively interacting with individuals from diverse backgrounds and belief systems. Therefore, healthcare professionals must demonstrate cultural competency by communicating effectively with patients while respecting their cultural values.

In today's healthcare landscape, having bilingual healthcare professionals who speak their patients' native language is a sign of respect. When healthcare facilities prioritize the need for care providers to speak the same language as their patients, it shows that those patients are valued. For example, Clínica Esperanza/Hope Clinic (CEHC) in Providence, Rhode Island, has developed the Advanced Navegante Training Program (ANTP) to address the growing demand for bilingual Community Health Workers (CHWs) in the healthcare sector. The ANTP, developed and taught by CEHC's own bilingual and bicultural CHWs, prepares community members to become certified CHWs who can provide patient navigation, lifestyle coaching, and professional medical interpretation services.

Bilingual and bicultural CHWs are highly sought after to serve as healthcare navigators, patient advocates, and medical interpreters in settings with a substantial Spanish-speaking patient population.

Overview of the book's content and structure

The "Learn Medical Spanish for Doctors and Nurses Workbook" is a complete tool designed to help medical professionals overcome language hurdles at work or in daily life in just 30 days. The workbook is essential for medical professionals because it gives them the most important Spanish vocabulary and phrases they need to communicate effectively with their Spanish-speaking patients.

This workbook was written by Elizabeth González Cueto, an accomplished medical doctor and M.Sc., who is fluent in English and French and is a native Spanish speaker. Her extensive educational background includes attending prestigious institutions such as National Polytechnic Institute in Mexico,

University of Tours in France, Hannover Medical School in Germany, and Autonomous University of Barcelona in Spain. Elizabeth has also completed research internships at the University of Oxford in the United Kingdom and at Mount Sinai Hospital in New York. With over four years of experience as a medical writer, reviewer, and editor for various global clients and companies, Elizabeth's expertise spans healthcare and scientific fields; her passion for medical writing makes her an exceptionally reliable source for medical Spanish education.

In addition, this workbook is full of real-life examples and exercises that medical professionals can use to improve their Spanish language skills, enhance their confidence, and build trust with Spanish-speaking patients. They can also learn the most important medical Spanish words and phrases, which will help them give better care to their patients.

One of the most important reasons to use this workbook is that it can help Spanish-speaking patients get better care and help patients and healthcare providers build trust, which can make patients more loyal.

The book is structured into 13 chapters, including an introduction and a conclusion. Each chapter focuses on a different aspect of medical Spanish, from basic vocabulary to cultural competence, with a range of activities, including grammar exercises and dialogues that simulate real-world medical situations.

In conclusion, "Learn Medical Spanish for Healthcare Professionals" is a great resource for medical professionals who want to improve their communication with Spanish-speaking patients. With its practical exercises, user-friendly layout, and expert author, this workbook is a great way for medical professionals to acquire the key Spanish terms and phrases they need to know to give their patients high-quality treatment. By learning medical Spanish, doctors and nurses may help their Spanish-speaking patients get the care they need to recover and move forward with their lives.

Guidelines for learning medical Spanish in 30 days

Purpose	The book aims to help healthcare professionals improve their Spanish language skills to communicate more effectively with Spanish-speaking patients in 30 days.
Audience	Intended for doctors, nurses, and other healthcare professionals who want to communicate more effectively with Spanish-speaking patients.
Use	The book can be used as a self-study guide or as part of a classroom course. Each chapter includes exercises and an answer key for self-assessment. Appendices offer additional resources, such as a glossary of medical terms, medical abbreviations, and a Spanish-English and English-Spanish medical dictionary.

Create a study plan	Break down the book's content into 30 days, assigning specific chapters to each day. Dedicate enough time to complete the exercises and review the answer keys for each chapter (find our suggested study plan at the end of this chapter).
Practice consistently	Consistency is key to learning Spanish quickly. Set aside a specific time each day to practice and maintain the schedule.
Start with the basics	Begin with the first two chapters, which cover Spanish basics and medical terminology. These lay the foundation for effective communication with Spanish-speaking patients.
Use flashcards	Use the digital flashcards included to reinforce learning. You can also create flashcards for each chapter's vocabulary and phrases and review them regularly. This will help you memorize the terms and recall them quickly when needed.
Practice with a partner	Practice conversations with a partner, such as a colleague or friend interested in learning medical Spanish. Role-playing exercises in the Additional Practice Exercises chapter are also great for interactive practice.
Use the glossary and dictionary	Use the glossary of medical Spanish terms and the Spanish-English and English-Spanish medical dictionary in the appendices to expand vocabulary and deepen understanding of medical terminology.
Use the answer key	Verify your exercise answers using the provided answer keys in each chapter to identify any areas where you need more practice.

Suggested study plan

The is a suggested study plan for learning medical Spanish in 4 weeks (30 days):

Week 1	
Day 1	Read the Introduction and Spanish Basics chapters. Complete exercises and review the answer key.
Day 2	Read the Basic Medical Terminology chapter. Complete exercises and review the answer key.
Day 3	Review the Spanish Basics chapter. Practice pronunciation and conversation skills.
Day 4	Review the Basic Medical Terminology chapter. Practice using medical terms in conversations.
Day 5	Read and complete exercises in the Anatomy and Physiology chapter.
Day 6-7	Review and practice the material covered in Week 1.

	Week 2	
Day 8	Read the Medical Procedures and Exams chapter. Complete exercises and review the answer key.	
Day 9	Read the Prescription and Medication chapter. Complete exercises and review the answer key.	
Day 10	Review the Medical Procedures and Exams chapter. Practice using vocabulary and giving instructions in Spanish.	
Day 11	Review the Prescription and Medication chapter. Practice discussing medication and dosage in Spanish.	
Day 12	Read and complete exercises in the Medical Emergencies chapter.	
Day 13-14	Review and practice the material covered in Week 2.	
	Week 3	
Day 15	Read the Enhancing Cultural Competence in Healthcare chapter. Complete exercises and review the answer key.	
Day 16	Read the Cultural Concepts in Hispanic Healthcare chapter. Complete exercises and review the answer key.	
Day 17	Review Enhancing Cultural Competence in Healthcare chapter. Practice using effective communication strategies in Spanish.	
Day 18	Review Cultural Concepts in Hispanic Healthcare chapter. Practice discussing traditional healing practices and common ailments in Spanish.	
Day 19	Complete additional practice exercises from Chapter IX.	
Day 20-21	Review and practice the material covered in Week 3.	
	Week 4	
Day 22	Review and practice material covered in previous weeks.	
Day 23	Review and practice material covered in previous weeks.	
Day 24	Review and practice material covered in previous weeks.	
Day 25	Complete additional practice exercises from Chapter IX.	
Day 26	Review and practice material covered in previous weeks.	
Day 27-28	Review and practice material covered in previous weeks.	
Day 29-30	Review and practice material covered in previous weeks. Use the appendices for reference as needed.	

We encourage you to adjust the plan to suit your needs and preferences. The goal is to cover all the material in the book within 4 weeks, allowing enough time for review and practice.

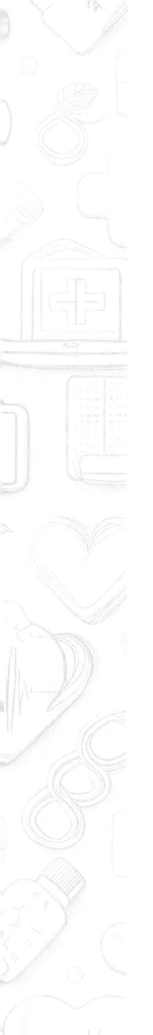

Chapter 2:
Spanish Basics

Cada idioma es un modo diferente de ver la vida.

Federico Fellini

As the healthcare industry becomes increasingly diverse, medical professionals must understand the Spanish language. This chapter provides a comprehensive overview of the Spanish language for medical professionals. We will begin with the basics of the Spanish alphabet, including pronunciation, and then move on to important medical phrases for greetings and introductions. Additionally, we will cover key medical vocabulary to help healthcare providers better communicate with their Spanish-speaking patients.

The alphabet

The Spanish alphabet consists of 27 letters, one more than the standard English alphabet. The additional letter is "ñ" (pronounced "enye"). While most letters are shared between Spanish and English, the pronunciation of some differs between the two languages. It is important to note that each letter in the Spanish alphabet consistently represents a specific sound. Previously, the Spanish alphabet included the letters "ch" and "ll" as distinct letters, making the total number of letters 29. However, as part of a reform to align with the international Latin alphabet, these letters are now treated as digraphs, not individual letters. As a result, words beginning with "ch" or "ll" are now categorized under the letters "c" and "i", respectively.

The Spanish sounds

Spanish is a phonetic language, which means that each letter has a distinct sound. Unlike English, Spanish is pronounced exactly as it is written. This characteristic underscores the importance of mastering Spanish sounds for effective communication

The Spanish vowel sounds

Spanish has five vowel sounds, which are "a," "e," "i," "o," and "u." In comparison with English, Spanish vowels always have the same sound and are pronounced in the same way. The pronunciation of each vowel is as follows:

Vowel	Pronunciation	Notes
A	Ah	as in "father"
E	Eh	as in "pet"
I	Ee	as in "me"
O	Oh	as in "go"
U	Oo	as in "cool"

The Spanish consonant sounds

Spanish has 22 consonant sounds. It is important to note that some consonant sounds are different from those in English. Therefore, practicing these sounds is necessary to ensure effective communication with Spanish-speaking patients. The Spanish consonant sounds are as follows:

Consonant	Pronunciation	Notes
B	"beh"	as in "be"
C	1. Before "a," "o," or "u," it's pronounced as a hard "k" 2. Before "e" or "i," it's pronounced as a soft "s" as in "cent."	1. Example: "casa" (kah-sah) 2. Example: "ciudad" (see-oo-dahd)
D	"deh"	as in "dog"
F	"efeh"	as in "fun"
G	"ge" 1. Before "a," "o," or "u," it's pronounced as a hard "g" sound, like the "g" in "go." 2. Before "e" or "i," it's pronounced as a soft "h" sound, like the "h" in "hot."	1. Example: "gato" (gah-toh) 2. Example: "gente" (hen-teh)
H	"hache" No sound	"h" is always silent in Spanish.
J	jota "h"	as in "hallelujah"
K	"Ka"	as in "kilogram"
L	"ele"	as in "love"

Consonant	Pronunciation	Notes
M	"eme"	as in "moon"
N	"ene"	as in "no"
Ñ	"ny" "gn"	as in "onion" or in "canyon"
P	"peh"	as in "pen"
Q	"cu"	as in "quit." However, when followed by an "e" or "i," it is always followed by a "u" and pronounced like the English "k" in "kite"
R	"ere o erre"	is pronounced with a rolling sound, similar to the Scottish "r"
S	"ese"	as in "sun"
T	"te"	as in "time"
V	"uve"	as in "victory"
W	"doble u", "doble ve" or "doble uve"	as in "Washington"
X	"equis"	as in "extra"
Y	"i griega o ye"	as in "yellow." However, when used as a vowel, it is pronounced like the English "ee" in "bee"
Z	"zeta"	as in "zebra"

Medical Spanish for greetings & introductions

Healthcare professionals should aim to make a good first impression when communicating with Spanish-speaking patients. Greetings and introductions play an important role in establishing rapport with patients. In addition, accents, words, and expressions change depending on the patient's Spanish-speaking. Below are some essential medical Spanish phrases for greetings and introductions:

Greeting	Spanish pronunciation	Meaning
Hola	oh-lah	Hello
¿Cómo está?	koh-moh ehs-tah	How are you? (Formal)
¿Cómo estás?	koh-moh ehs-tahs	How are you? (Informal)
¿Cómo se siente?	koh-moh seh syen-teh?	How do you feel? (Formal)

Greeting	Spanish pronunciation	Meaning
¿Cómo te sientes?	koh-moh teh syen-tehs?	How do you feel? (Informal)
Bien, gracias	bee-ehn, grah-see-yahs	Well, thank you
¿Cómo se llama?	koh-moh seh yah-mah	What is your name? (Formal)
¿Cómo te llamas?	koh-moh teh yah-mahs	What is your name? (Informal)
Me llamo	meh yah-moh	My name is
Encantado/a	ehn-kahn-tah-doh/dah	Nice to meet you (male/female)
Mucho gusto	moo-choh goo-stoh	Nice to meet you
Soy un/a doctor/a	soy oon/ah dohk-tohr/ah	I am a doctor (male/female)
Soy un/a enfermero/a	soy oon/oon-ah en-fer-meh-ro/rah	I am a nurse (male/female)
¿Habla inglés?	ah-blah een-glehs	Do you speak English?
Necesito su ayuda	neh-seh-see-toh soo ah-yoo-dah	I need your help
¿Dónde está el hospital?	dohn-deh ehs-tah ehl oh-spee-tahl	Where is the hospital?
¿Cómo puedo ayudarle?	koh-moh pweh-doh ah-yoo-dahr-leh	How can I help you? (Formal)
¿Cómo puedo ayudarte?	koh-moh pweh-doh ah-yoo-dahr-teh	How can I help you? (Informal)

Notes:

The phrases "¿Cómo está?" and "¿Cómo estás?" both translate to "How are you?" in English, but they have grammatical differences in Spanish.

- "¿Cómo está?" is in the third person singular, which is used to address someone formally or respectfully. This form is appropriate when addressing someone you do not know or someone of higher status, such as an elderly person, a professor, or a superior at work. *This language form is typically used in formal settings such as doctor's consultations, as it conveys respect.* *

- "¿Cómo estás?" is in the second person singular, which is used to address someone informally or casually. This form is appropriate when addressing someone you know well, someone of the same age or social status, or someone younger than you.

The phrases "¿Cómo se llama?" and "¿Cómo te llamas?" both translate to "What's your name?" in English, but they have grammatical differences in Spanish.

- "¿Cómo se llama?" is in the third person singular, which is used to address someone formally or respectfully. This form is appropriate when addressing someone you do not know or someone of higher status, such as an elderly person, a professor, or a superior at work.

- "¿Cómo te llamas?" is in the second person singular, which is used to address someone informally or casually. This form is appropriate when addressing someone you know well, someone of the same age or social status, or someone younger than you.

In Spanish, the words "doctor" and "doctora" both mean "doctor" in English, but they have gender differences.

- "Doctor" is the masculine form and is used to address a male doctor or a female doctor when addressing a group that includes both men and women.

  For example: El doctor González es muy amable (Doctor González is very kind).

- "Doctora" is the feminine form and is used to address a female doctor.

- For example: La doctora Ramírez es una excelente cirujana (Doctor Ramírez is an excellent surgeon).

Moreover, the words "médico" and "médica" both translate to "medic" in English. The difference lies in their gender: "médico" is used for a male doctor, while "médica" is used for a female doctor.

- For example: Soy el/la médico/médica que le atenderá hoy (I am the attending physician for you today)

- Additional examples:

  - Masculine: enfermero (nurse), farmacéutico (pharmacist), trabajador social, (social worker), nutriólogo (nutritionist), camillero (stretcher-bearer), psicólogo (psychologist)

  - Femenine: enfermera (nurse), farmacéutica (pharmacist), trabajadora social (social worker), nutrilóga (nutritionist), camillera (stretcher-bearer), psicóloga (psychologist)

Regarding the inclusion of the pronoun "elle" to refer to the subject of neutral gender in Spanish:

People who identify as non-binary —neither male nor female— advocate for the use of the pronoun "elle" instead of "él" or "ella" and the ending -e. The following are examples:

- Elle está cansade (They is tired)

- Trabajadore social (Social worker)

When addressing someone in Spanish, it's essential to use the correct gender, as it shows respect and consideration for their gender identity.

Practical tips for healthcare providers:

- Be mindful of pronouns: Always ask patients their preferred pronouns and address them accordingly.

- Use professional interpreters: Use professional interpreters when language barriers are present to ensure clear and accurate communication.

- Cultural sensitivity training: Engage in ongoing cultural competence training to better understand the diverse backgrounds of Spanish-speaking patients.

- Patient-centered communication: Use open-ended questions and active listening to understand patients' health beliefs and practices.

Incorporating these practices enables healthcare providers to deliver more effective and respectful care to their Spanish-speaking patients.

Useful phrases

Now, let's practice some conversations using the phrases we learned:

Conversation 1:

	Spanish		English
Doctor	¡Hola! ¿Cómo está?	Doctor	Hello! How are you?
Paciente	¡Hola! Bien gracias, ¿y usted?	Patient	Hi! I'm good, and you?
Doctor	Estoy bien, gracias. ¿Cómo se llama?	Doctor	I'm good, thank you. What is your name?
Paciente	Me llamo Ana.	Patient	My name is Ana.
Doctor	Encantado, Ana. El día de hoy seré su médico tratante. ¿En qué puedo ayudarle?	Doctor	Nice to meet you, Ana. Today I will be your attending physician. How can I help you?
Paciente	Vengo por que tengo mucho dolor de cabeza desde ayer y a pesar de que tomé medicamentos el dolor no mejora.	Patient	I am here because I've had headache since yesterday, and even though I've taken medication, the pain is not getting better.
Doctor	Claro, vamos a revisarla. Por favor, sígame.	Doctor	Sure, let's check it. Please, follow me.

Conversation 2:

	Spanish		English
Enfermera	¡Hola! ¿Cómo está?	Nurse	Hello! How are you?
Paciente	Hola, estoy un poco nervioso.	Patient	Hi, I'm a little nervous.
Enfermera	¿Cómo se llama?	Nurse	What is your name?
Paciente	Me llamo Miguel.	Patient	My name is Miguel.
Enfermera	Mucho gusto, Miguel. Soy su enfermera, ¿habla inglés?	Nurse	Nice to meet you, Miguel. I am your nurse, do you speak English?
Paciente	Sí, hablo inglés.	Patient	Yes, I speak English.
Enfermera	Perfecto. ¿Dónde le duele?	Nurse	Perfect. Where is the pain?
Paciente	Me duele el estómago.	Patient	My stomach hurts.

Enfermera	Entiendo. Vamos a tomarle la temperatura y medir la presión arterial para ver cómo se encuentra.	Nurse	I understand. Let's take your temperature and measure your blood pressure to see how you're doing.

Spanish		English	
Doctor	¡Hola! ¿Cómo está?	Doctor	Hello! How are you?
Paciente	Hola, no me siento bien.	Patient	Hi, I don't feel well.
Doctor	¿Cómo se llama?	Doctor	What is your name?
Paciente	Me llamo Juan.	Patient	My name is Juan.
Doctor	Encantado, Juan. ¿Por qué no se siente bien?	Doctor	Nice to meet you, Juan. Why don't you feel well?
Paciente	Me duele la garganta y tengo fiebre.	Patient	My throat hurts and I have a fever.
Doctor	Entiendo, ¿habla inglés?	Doctor	I understand, do you speak English?
Paciente	No mucho.	Patient	Not much.
Doctor	No hay problema. La enfermera y yo hablamos español, podemos asistirlo y responder sus dudas. Voy a examinarlo para ver qué está sucediendo.	Doctor	No problem. The nurse and I speak Spanish, we can assist you and answer your questions. I will examine you to see what is going on.

The best way to learn and retain Spanish

Learning Spanish can be challenging, especially if you have never been exposed to the language or have interacted with Spanish speakers. However, as a healthcare professional, speaking Spanish can be a valuable asset that can help you communicate better with your patients and provide better care. Here are some tips to help you learn and retain Spanish effectively:

Set goals	Do you want to be able to understand basic medical terms and phrases, or do you want to be able to have full conversations with your patients? Setting clear goals will help you focus your learning efforts and track your progress.
Use multiple Resources	Use a combination of textbooks, workbooks, podcasts, cards, notes, figures, drawings, online resources, and apps to help you learn Spanish. Each resource offers a different approach to learning and reinforces the concepts you are studying.

Practice regularly	Set aside time each day to practice your Spanish, even if it's just for a few minutes. Practice with known Spanish speakers—whether they are family, friends, or colleagues. Consistency is key, and regular practice can help you retain what you've learned and improve your skills.
Inmmerse yourself	Immerse yourself in Spanish culture by listening to Spanish music, watching Spanish movies and TV shows, listening to podcasts and reading Spanish books and news articles. Social media also provides opportunities to follow medical Spanish influencers and learn from their informative content in Spanish.
Speak and listen	Language learning involves both speaking and listening. Practice speaking with native speakers or other healthcare professionals who are learning Spanish to improve your pronunciation and fluency. Gradually, you can begin using a few words with your patients. Additionally, listening to Spanish conversations or recordings can help you improve your comprehension and vocabulary.
Use mnemonics	Mnemonics are memory aids that can help you remember new words and phrases. Create your own mnemonics or use existing ones to help you remember medical terms and phrases in Spanish. For example, to remember the Spanish word for "stomach," you could use the mnemonic "ESTO-mago" or "fiebre" for "fever," which sounds similar to the English word.
Find medical anglicisms in Spanish	Medical anglicisms are English words that are adopted into Spanish, often with slight modifications in spelling or pronunciation. These terms are frequently used in the medical field due to the global influence of English-speaking countries on medicine and healthcare. -----For example, the term "check-up" is translated as "chequeo," referring to a general medical examination or routine health check. The word "test" remains "test" in both languages. Similarly, "stress" becomes "estrés" in Spanish, describing psychological or physical stress.
Seek feedback	Seek feedback from native speakers or other healthcare professionals on your pronunciation and speaking skills. Constructive feedback can help you identify areas for improvement and refine your language skills.
Use the glossary and dictionary	Use the glossary of medical Spanish terms and the Spanish-English and English-Spanish medical dictionary in the appendices to expand vocabulary and deepen understanding of medical terminology.
Use the answer key	Verify your exercise answers using the provided answer keys in each chapter to identify any areas where you need more practice.

Key takeaways

In this chapter, we covered the basics of the Spanish language, focusing on the Spanish alphabet and sounds. We also introduced essential medical Spanish phrases for greetings and introductions. The key takeaways from this chapter are:

- The Spanish alphabet has 27 letters, including one additional letter "ñ".
- Spanish is a phonetic language, which means that each letter has a distinct sound.
- Spanish incorporates five vowel sounds and 22 consonant sounds.
- Mastering the basic Spanish sounds is fundamental to communicate effectively in medical settings.
- Key medical Spanish phrases for greetings and introductions include "Hola," "¿Cómo está?" and "Soy un(a) doctor(a)".

Exercises

Exercise 1

Write the Spanish pronunciation for the following English words:

No.	English	Spanish
1	Father	
2	Pet	
3	Me	
4	Boat	
5	Blue	

Exercise 2

Write the English pronunciation for the following Spanish words:

No.	English	Spanish
1	Perro	
2	Gato	
3	Médico	
4	Hospital	
5	Enfermera	

Exercise 3

Complete the following sentences in Spanish:

¿_____ es su nombre? (What is your name?)

_____ es un/a doctor/a. (He/She is a doctor/nurse.)

¿_____ está el hospital? (Where is the hospital?)

¿_____ puedo ayudarle? (How can I help you?)

Mucho _____. (Nice to meet you.)

Answer key

Exercise 1

Write the Spanish pronunciation for the following English words:

No.	English	Spanish
1	Father	padre (pah-dreh)
2	Pet	mascota (mahs-koh-tah)
3	Me	yo (yoh)
4	Boat	barco (bar-koh)
5	Blue	azul (ah-sool)

Exercise 2

Write the English pronunciation for the following Spanish words:

No.	English	Spanish
1	Perro	dog (peh-roh)
2	Gato	cat (gah-toh)
3	Médico	doctor (meh-dee-koh)
4	Hospital	hospital (oh-spee-tahl)
5	Enfermera	nurse (en-fehr-meh-rah)

Exercise 3

Complete the following sentences in Spanish:

¿Cuál es su nombre? (What is your name?)

Él/Ella es un(a) doctor(a). (He/She is a doctor/nurse.)

¿Dónde está el hospital? (Where is the hospital?)

¿Cómo puedo ayudarle? (How can I help you?)

Mucho gusto. (Nice to meet you.)

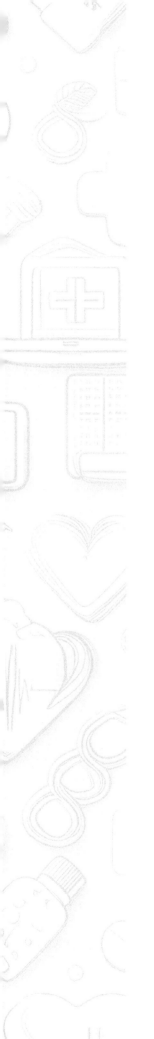

Chapter 3:
Basic Medical Terminology

La medicina no es solo una ciencia, sino también el arte de dejar que nuestra individualidad se relacione con la de nuestros pacientes.

William Osler

Introduction to medical terminology in Spanish

Medical terminology is an essential part of healthcare, and being proficient in it is crucial for healthcare professionals who interact with Spanish-speaking patients. In this chapter, we will introduce medical terminology in Spanish, helping you communicate effectively with your Spanish-speaking patients.

As mentioned in the introduction, knowing the proper medical terms in Spanish is particularly important when communicating with patients who may not speak English fluently. Language barriers can lead to misunderstandings, which can affect patient care and outcomes. By mastering essential medical terms and phrases in Spanish, healthcare professionals can ensure clear and effective with their Spanish-speaking patients.

This chapter covers the most common medical terms and phrases in Spanish, including body parts, symptoms, diseases, and treatments. We will also discuss the proper use of these terms in a medical context to ensure accurate communication. By the end of this chapter, you will have a better understanding of medical terminology in Spanish, enhancing your ability to provide high-quality care to Spanish-speaking patients.

In addition to benefiting healthcare professionals, this chapter may also be useful for students studying medical terminology or anyone interested in learning more about the Spanish language in a medical context. Whether you are just starting to learn Spanish or have been speaking it for years, this chapter will provide you with a solid foundation in medical terminology.

Common medical terms and phrases in Spanish

Medical terminology is a specialized language used in the healthcare industry. Knowing common medical terms and phrases in Spanish will help you understand patient needs, provide instructions, and explain medical procedures. Here are some of the most common medical terms and phrases in Spanish:

Medical terms in Spanish	Medical terms in English
Corazón	Heart
Riñón	Kidney
Pulmón	Lung
Hígado	Liver
Cerebro	Brain
Sangre	Blood
Hueso	Bone
Cáncer	Cancer
Infección	Infection
Diabetes	Diabetes
Enfermedad	Disease
Fiebre	Fever
Dolor	Pain
Presión arterial	Blood pressure
Vacuna	Vaccine
Tratamiento	Treatment
Antibiótico	Antibiotic
Inflamación	Inflammation
Radiografía	X-ray
Nutrición	Nutrition
Paciente	Patient
Terapia	Therapy
Síntomas	Symptoms
Salud	Health
Cirugía	Surgery

Medical terms in Spanish	Medical terms in English
Emergencia	Emergency
Dosis	Dose
Medicamento	Medication
Venas	Veins
Músculo	Muscle
Hormona	Hormone
Terapeuta	Therapist
Especialista	Specialist
Epidemia	Epidemic
Contagio	Contagion
Medicina	Medicine
Órganos	Organs
Enfermero(a)	Nurse
Deshidratación	Dehydration
Asma	Asthma
Infarto	Heart attack
Anestesia	Anesthesia
Trasplante	Transplant
Hemorragia	Hemorrhage
Psiquiatría	Psychiatry
Traumatismo	Trauma
Síndrome	Syndrome
Virus	Virus
Quimioterapia	Chemotherapy
Radioterapia	Radiation therapy
Ojos	Eyes
Convulsión	Seizure
Hospitalización	Hospitalization
Anticonceptivos	Birth control
Emergencia médica	Medical emergency

Medical terms in Spanish	Medical terms in English
Congénito	Congenital
Seguro médico	Health insurance

Pronunciation and spelling rules for medical Spanish

Pronunciation is a fundamental component of communication, and it is especially important in the healthcare industry. Knowing the correct pronunciation of medical terminology in Spanish will help you communicate more effectively with your Spanish-speaking patients. Here are some pronunciation and spelling rules for medical Spanish:

- The letter "J" in Spanish is pronounced like the "h" in "hot."
  For instance, "juego" (game) is pronounced "hweh-go" and the word "jirafa" (giraffe) is pronounced "hee-rah-fah".

- The pronunciation of "G" in Spanish varies based on the following letter. Before "e" or "i," it sounds like the "h" in "hot." Conversely, before "a," "o," or "u," it resembles "g" in "go."
  For example, "ginecólogo" (gynecologist) is pronounced "hee-neh-koh-loh-goh."

- Similarly, "C" in Spanish changes its sound depending on the following letter. Before "e" or "i," it is pronounced like the "s" in "sit." When it precedes "a," "o," or "u," it sounds like the "k" in "kite."
  For example, "cirugía" (surgery) is pronounced "see-roo-hee-yah."

- In Spanish, the letter "H" is always silent.
  For instance, "hígado" (liver) is pronounced "ee-gah-doh."

- The letters "LL" and "Y" have similar sounds in Spanish. For example:

  ⊙ callado (quiet/silent)

  ⊙ cayado (staff/cane)

  ⊙ cayado aórtico (aortic arch)

  Note that in some Spanish-speaking countries, such as Argentina and Uruguay, the "LL" sound is pronounced like a "sh" sound, while in others, such as Spain and Mexico, it is pronounced like a "y" sound. This can sometimes lead to regional variations in spelling.

- Accents are used in Spanish to indicate where the stress falls on a word.
  For example, the word "médico" (doctor) is stressed on the third-to-last syllable and has an accent mark on the "e". On the other hand, the word "medicó" (he/she treated medically) is stressed on the last syllable, indicated by the accent on the "o".

By following these pronunciation and spelling rules, you will be better equipped to communicate with your Spanish-speaking patients and colleagues in a clear and effective manner.

Examples of conversations between doctors/nurses and patients

Mastering medical terminology is essential, but being able to communicate it effectively with patients is just as important. Here are some examples of interactions between healthcare professionals and patients:

Conversation 1:

	Spanish		English
Doctor	Hola, ¿cómo se siente hoy?	Doctor	Hi, how are you feeling today?
Paciente	No me siento bien. Tengo fiebre y dolor en el pecho.	Patient	I don't feel well. I have a fever and chest pain.
Doctor	¿Ha tenido problemas en el corazón antes?	Doctor	Have you had any heart problems before?
	Spanish		**English**
Paciente	Sí, tengo la presión alta.	Patient	es, I have high blood pressure.
Doctor	En este caso le tomaremos la presión arterial y después usaré el estetoscopio para examinar su corazón.	Doctor	In this case, we will measure your blood pressure and then I will use the stethoscope to examine your heart.
Paciente	Entiendo, doctor.	Patient	I understand, doctor.
Doctor	Entiendo, necesito hacerle una revisión general, un electrocardiograma, y una radiografía de tórax para ver qué podría estar causando el dolor en su pecho. Después podremos decidir mejor su tratamiento. ¿Está de acuerdo?	Doctor	I understand, I need to perform a general check-up, an electrocardiogram, and a chest x-ray to see what might be causing your chest pain. Then we can determine the best treatment for you. Do you agree

Conversation 2:

	Spanish		English
Enfermera	Hola, ¿cómo se siente hoy?	Nurse	Hi, how are you feeling today?
Paciente	Me duele mucho el riñón.	Patient	My kidney hurts a lot.
Enfermera	¿Ha estado tomando sus medicamentos para la infección del riñón?	Nurse	Have you been taking your medications for the kidney infection?

	Spanish		English
Paciente	No, olvidé tomarlos ayer.	Patient	No, I forgot to take them yesterday.
Enfermera	Es muy importante que tome sus medicamentos para que pueda recuperarse rápidamente.	Nurse	It's very important that you take your medication so you can recover quickly.

Conversation 3:

	Spanish		English
Doctor	Hola, ¿cómo ha estado desde la última vez que nos vimos?	Doctor	Hi, how have you been since the last time we saw each other?
Paciente	Me he sentido bien en general, pero todavía tengo dolores de cabeza y mareos.	Patient	I've been feeling good overall, but I still have headaches and dizziness.
Doctor	¿Se ha sentido deprimido o ansioso recientemente?	Doctor	Have you been feeling depressed or anxious recently?
Paciente	Sí, me he sentido muy ansioso últimamente.	Patient	Yes, I've been feeling very anxious lately.
Doctor	Le voy a dar una interconsulta con un especialista en psiquiatría para que evalúe su caso.	Doctor	I will give you a referral to a psychiatric specialist to evaluate your case.

Conversation 4:

	Spanish		English
Enfermera	Hola, ¿cómo ha estado desde su cirugía?	Nurse	Hi, how have you been since your surgery?
Paciente	Me he estado recuperando bien, pero todavía tengo dolores en los huesos y los músculos.	Patient	I've been recovering well, but I'm still experiencing discomfort in my bones and muscles.
Enfermera	¿Ha estado tomando sus medicamentos para el dolor?	Nurse	Have you been taking your pain medication?
Paciente	Sí, pero no parecen estar funcionando tan bien como antes.	Patient	Yes, but they don't seem to be working as well as before.
Enfermera	Puedo hablar con el médico para que le recete un medicamento diferente si es necesario.	Nurse	I can talk to the doctor to prescribe a different medication for you if needed.

Key takeaways

- Fluency in Spanish is required for effective communication with Spanish-speaking patients among healthcare professionals.

- Language barriers can lead to misunderstandings that impact patient care and outcomes. A robust understanding of essential medical terms and phrases in Spanish ensures clear and effective communication.

- This chapter covers the most common medical terms and phrases in Spanish, including body parts, symptoms, diseases, and treatments.

- Correct pronunciation is an important component of communication, it enables healthcare professionals to communicate more effectively with their Spanish-speaking patients.

Exercises

Exercise 1

Write the Spanish equivalent for the following English medical terms:

No.	English	Spanish
1	Heart	
2	Kidney	
3	Lung	
4	Liver	
5	Brain	
6	Blood	
7	Bone	
8	Cancer	
9	Infection	
10	Diabetes	

Exercise 2

Match the following Spanish medical terms with their corresponding English equivalents:

No.	English	Spanish
1	Fiebre	Fever
2	Presión arterial	Antibiotic

3	Vacuna	Treatment
4	Tratamiento	Blood pressure
5	Antibiótico	Vaccine

Exercise 3

Choose the correct pronunciation of the following medical terms:

1. Corazón

    a. ko-rah-zon

    b. ko-rah-thohn

    c. ko-rah-sohn

2. Ginecólogo

    a. gih-neh-koh-loh-goh

    b. gee-neh-koh-loh-goh

    c. hee-neh-koh-loh-goh

3. Cirugía

    a. see-roo-gyah

    b. see-roo-hee-yah

    c. kee-roo-gyah

Exercise 4

Fill in the blank with the correct pronunciation of the medical term:

Spanish word	Pronunciation
Hígado	ee-gah-_____
Enfermedad	en-fer-meh-_____
Hemorragia	eh-moh-rah-_____

Answer key

Exercise 1

No.	English	Spanish
1	Heart	Corazón
2	Kidney	Riñón
3	Lung	Pulmón
4	Liver	Hígado
5	Brain	Cerebro
6	Blood	Sangre
7	Bone	Hueso
8	Cancer	Cáncer
9	Infection	Infección
10	Diabetes	Diabetes

Exercise 2

Match the following Spanish medical terms with their corresponding English meanings:

No.	English	Spanish
1	Fiebre	Fever
2	Presión arterial	Blood pressure
3	Vacuna	Vaccine
4	Tratamiento	Treatment
5	Antibiótico	Antibiotic

Exercise 3

1. c. ko-rah-sohn

2. a. gee-neh-koh-loh-goh

3. b. see-roo-hee-yah

Exercise 4

Spanish word	Pronunciation
Hígado	ee-gah-__doh___
Enfermedad	en-fer-meh-__dahd____
Hemorragia	eh-moh-rah-_ hee-ah_

A solid grasp medical terminology in Spanish is indispensable for healthcare professionals to provide accurate and efficient care to Spanish-speaking patients. This chapter has introduced essential medical terms and phrases, along with guidelines for pronunciation and spelling, and examples of dialogue between healthcare providers and patients. Continuous practice and improvement of your medical Spanish skills can lead to better communication and improved health outcomes for Spanish-speaking patients.

BOOK

02

Spanish Medical Communication: Anatomy, Procedures, Prescription, and Emergencies

Fluency for Better Care: Discovering Medical Spanish Language, Human Body, and Practices!

Book 2 Description

Welcome to the second part of our transformative series, 'Medical Terminology, Anatomy, and Procedures.' As a dedicated healthcare professional, your journey to becoming a proficient Spanish speaker continues, propelling you toward delivering exceptional patient care and fostering genuine connections.

This comprehensive guide navigates the intricacies of medical terminology in Spanish. You will learn common medical terms, phrases, and pronunciations specific to medical contexts. From basic anatomy and physiology terms to in-depth knowledge of the body's systems and apparatuses, we've curated everything you need.

Clear communication is especially important during procedures and examinations. This book provides you with the vocabulary needed to conduct medical procedures and exams in Spanish, along with essential patient consultation phrases and instructions.

Moreover, we understand the significance of medication management. We've compiled a comprehensive list of Spanish terms related to prescriptions and medications. You'll confidently discuss allergies, side effects, explain dosage, and communicate medication information accurately.

Throughout the book, real-life examples of conversations between medical professionals and patients reinforce your learning and practical application of medical Spanish Join us as we explore and deepen your understanding of medical communication in Spanish.

Chapter 1:
Anatomy and Physiology

La belleza del cuerpo es muchas veces indicio de la hermosura del alma.

Miguel de Cervantes

Basic anatomy and physiology terms in Spanish

Mastering basic anatomy and physiology terms in Spanish is essential for effective communication with patients, which is foundational to delivering quality healthcare as healthcare professionals in today's diverse society. This knowledge breaks down language barriers, enabling patients to understand their medical conditions and treatment plans. This chapter aims to equip healthcare professionals with the necessary vocabulary to communicate with Spanish-speaking patients confidently. We will delve into the various body systems and their functions, explore common medical conditions related to each system, and provide practical examples of conversations between healthcare professionals and patients. By the end of this chapter, you will have a solid foundation in medical Spanish, enabling you to provide better care to your Spanish-speaking patients.

For effective communication with Spanish-speaking patients, familiarity with basic anatomy and physiology terms in Spanish is crucial. Here are key terms to remember:

Spanish	English
Anatomía	Anatomy
Fisiología	Physiology
Sistema nervioso	Nervous system
Sistema cardiovascular	Cardiovascular system
Sistema respiratorio	Respiratory system
Sistema digestivo	Digestive system
Sistema endocrino	Endocrine system
Sistema muscular	Muscular system

Spanish	English
Sistema óseo	Skeletal system
Sistema linfático	Lymphatic system
Sistema urinario	Urinary system
Sistema reproductor	Reproductive system
Tejido	Tissue
Célula	Cell
Glóbulo rojo	Red blood cell
Glóbulo blanco	White blood cell
Plaqueta	Platelet
Epitelio	Epithelium
Cartílago	Cartilage
Hueso	Bone
Músculo	Muscle
Ligamento	Ligament
Tendón	Tendon
Articulación	Joint
Neurona	Neuron
Sinapsis	Synapse
Cerebro	Brain
Médula espinal	Spinal cord
Ganglio	Ganglion
Nervio	Nerve
Corazón	Heart
Vena	Vein
Arteria	Artery
Capilar	Capillary
Pulmón	Lung
Tráquea	Trachea
Bronquio	Bronchus
Diafragma	Diaphragm

Spanish	English
Estómago	Stomach
Hígado	Liver
Páncreas	Pancreas
Intestino delgado	Small intestine
Intestino grueso (colon)	Large intestine (colon)
Vesícula biliar	Gallbladder
Glándula tiroides	Thyroid gland
Glándula suprarrenal	Adrenal gland
Glándula pituitaria	Pituitary gland
Riñón	Kidney
Vejiga	Bladder
Ovario	Ovary

Body parts and their functions

Below are some key body parts and their functions, organized by systems and apparatuses:

Skeletal system: Supports and structures the body through bones, ligaments, and cartilage.

1. hueso: bone
2. cartílago: cartilage
3. tendón: tendon
4. ligamento: ligament
5. músculo: muscle
6. vertebras: vertebrae
7. cráneo: skull
8. articulación: joint
9. médula ósea: bone marrow
10. fémur: femur

Muscular system: Responsible for movement and posture through muscles and tendons.

1. músculo: muscle
2. sistema muscular esquelético: skeletal muscular system

3. músculos lisos: smooth muscles

4. músculos cardíacos: cardiac muscles

5. masa muscular: muscle mass

6. contracción muscular: muscle contraction

7. fibra muscular: muscle fiber

8. tono muscular: muscle tone

9. miopatía: myopathy

10. miembro inferior: lower limb

Nervous system: Controls and coordinates the body's functions and responses to stimuli through the brain, spinal cord, and nerves.

1. cerebro: brain

2. médula espinal: spinal cord

3. nervios: nerves

4. neuronas: neurons

5. sistemas sensoriales: sensory systems

6. sistema nervioso autónomo: autonomic nervous system

7. neurotransmisores: neurotransmitters

8. sinapsis: synapses

9. corteza cerebral: cerebral cortex

10. sistema nervioso periférico: peripheral nervous system

Circulatory system: Transports blood, nutrients, and oxygen throughout the body through the heart, blood vessels, and blood.

1. corazón: heart

2. arteria: artery

3. vena: vein

4. capilar: capillary

5. sistema cardiovascular: cardiovascular system

6. plasma sanguíneo: blood plasma

7. globulos rojos (eritrocitos): red blood cells (erythrocytes)

8. globulos blancos (leucocitos): white blood cells (leukocytes)

9. hemoglobina: hemoglobin

10. circulación sanguínea: blood circulation

Respiratory system: Facilitates the exchange of gases (oxygen and carbon dioxide) between the body and the environment.

1. pulmón: lung

2. tráquea: trachea

3. bronquio: bronchus

4. alvéolo: alveolus

5. diafragma: diaphragm

6. vía aérea: airway

7. intercambio gaseoso: gas exchange

8. respiración: breathing

9. capacidad pulmonar: lung capacity

10. cavidad nasal: nasal cavity

Digestive system: Breaks down food into smaller molecules for the body's absorption and to eliminates waste products.

1. boca: mouth

2. esófago: esophagus

3. estómago: stomach

4. recto: rectum

5. ano: anus

6. hígado: liver

7. vesícula biliar: gallbladder

8. páncreas: pancreas

9. intestino delgado: small intestine

10. intestino grueso: large intestine

Urinary system: Its function is to remove waste products from the blood and to regulate fluid and electrolyte balance in the body.

1. riñón: kidney

2. uretra: urethra

3. vejiga: bladder

4. tracto urinario: urinary tract

5. filtración renal: renal filtration

6. orina: urine

7. sistema excretor: excretory system

8. regulación del equilibrio ácido-base: regulation of acid-base balance

9. sistema renina-angiotensina-aldosterona: renin-angiotensin-aldosterone system

10. sistema urinario masculino/femenino: male/female urinary system.

Reproductive system: Produces and transports gametes (sperm and eggs) to facilitate reproduction.

1. ovario: ovary

2. útero: uterus

3. vagina: vagina

4. pene: penis

5. testículo: testicle

6. epidídimo: epididymis

7. próstata: prostate

8. glándulas de Bartolino: Bartholin's glands

9. células de Leydig: Leydig cells

10. trompas de Falopio: Fallopian tubes

Endocrine system: Regulates bodily functions such as growth, metabolism, and reproduction.

1. glándula: gland

2. hormonas: hormones

3. hipotálamo: hypothalamus

4. pituitaria: pituitary gland

5. tiroides: thyroid gland

6. paratiroides: parathyroid gland

7. páncreas: pancreas

8. adrenalina: adrenaline

9. glucagon: glucagon

10. insulina: insulin

Integumentary system: Protects the body from external damage and regulates body temperature.

1. piel: skin

2. cabello: hair

3. uñas: nails

4. glándulas sudoríparas: sweat glands

5. glándulas sebáceas: sebaceous glands

6. estrato córneo: stratum corneum

7. epidermis: epidermis

8. dermis: dermis

9. hipodermis: hypodermis

10. termorregulación: thermoregulation

Lymphatic system: Defends the body from infection and disease by transporting immune cells and filtering harmful substances from the blood.

1. linfocitos: lymphocytes

2. ganglios linfáticos: lymph nodes

3. sistema linfático: the lymphatic system

4. vasos linfáticos: lymphatic vessels

5. bazo: spleen

6. amígdalas: tonsils

7. timo: thymus

8. linfoma: lymphoma

9. inflamación linfática: lymphadenitis

10. líquido linfático: lymphatic fluid

Visual system: Processes visual information from the environment and transmits it to the brain for interpretation.

1. eye: ojo

2. córnea: cornea

3. retina: retina

4. párpados: eyelids

5. cristalino: lens

6. pupilas: pupils

7. mácula: macula

8. campo visual: visual field

9. reflejo pupilar: pupillary reflex

10. agudeza visual: visual acuity

Spanish / English diagrams of the human body systems and apparatuses

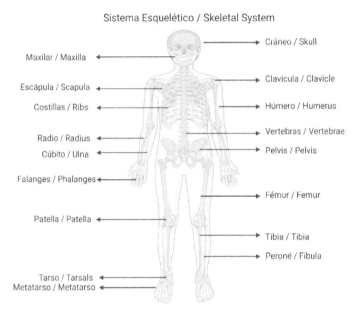

The skeletal system, anterior view, Created with BioRender.com

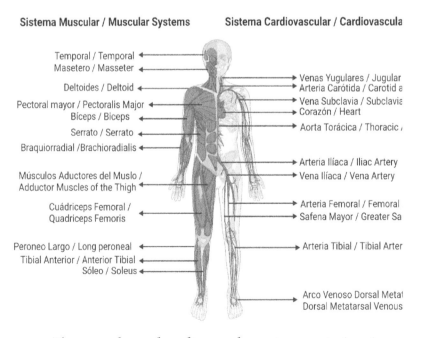

The muscular and cardiovascular systems, anterior view.
Created with BioRender.com

Sistema Digestivo / Digestive System

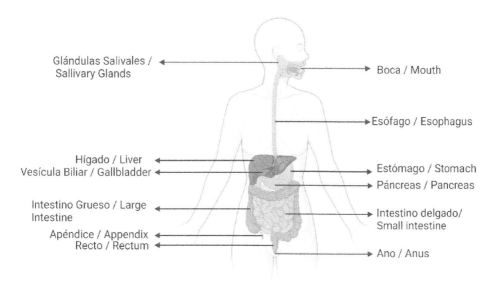

The digestive system, anterior view, Created with BioRender.com

Sitema Respiratorio / Respiratory System

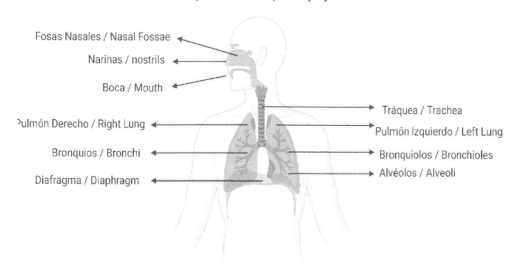

The respiratory system, anterior view, Created with BioRender.com

Anatomía del Ojo Humano/ Anatomy of the Human Eye

Músculo ciliar/ Ciliary muscle

Cámara posterior/ Posterior chamber

Córnea/ Cornea

Iris/ Iris

Pupila/ Pupil

Humor acuoso/ Aqueous humor

Cristalino/ Lens

Fibras zonulares/ Zonule fibers

Esclerótica/ Sclera

Coroides/ Choroid

Fóvea/ Fovea

Disco óptico/ Optic disk

Nervio óptico y vasos retinianos/ Optic nerve and retinal vessels

Humor vítreo/ Vitreous humor

Retina/ Retina

Anatomy of the eye, lateral view, Created with BioRender.com

Medical conditions and diseases related to the body's systems

Now that you have a solid understanding of the various systems of the human body, it is important to understand the different medical conditions and diseases that can affect these systems. Below, you will find some of the most common medical conditions and diseases encountered by healthcare professionals, along with their corresponding Spanish terms:

Respiratory system

1. Asthma (asma)

2. Chronic obstructive pulmonary disease or COPD (Enfermedad Pulmonar Obstructiva Crónica or EPOC)

3. Pneumonia (neumonía)

4. Bronchitis (bronquitis)

5. Emphysema (enfisema)

6. Tuberculosis (tuberculosis)

7. Pulmonary fibrosis (fibrosis pulmonar)

8. Lung cancer (cáncer de pulmón)

9. Cystic fibrosis (fibrosis quística)

10. Pleural effusion (derrame pleural)

Cardiovascular System

1. Hypertension (hipertensión)

2. Coronary artery disease (enfermedad arterial coronaris)

3. Heart failure (insuficiencia cardiaca)

4. Myocardial infarction (infarto de miocardio)

5. Arrhythmia (arritmia)

6. Hypertrophic cardiopathy (cardiopatía hipertrófica)

7. Atherosclerosis (aterosclerosis)

8. Cardiomyopathy (miocardiopatía)

9. Pericarditis (pericarditis)

10. Endocarditis (endocarditis)

Digestive system

1. Gastroesophageal reflux disease or GERD (enfermedad por reflujo gastroesofágico or ERGE)

2. Irritable bowel syndrome or IBS (síndrome de intestino irritable or SII)

3. Hepatitis (hepatitis)

4. Cirrhosis (cirrosis)

5. Gallstones (cálculos biliares)

6. Peptic ulcer (úlcera péptica)

7. Diarrhea (diarrea)

8. Diverticulitis (diverticulitis)

9. Constipation (constipación)

10. Crohn's disease (enfermedad de Crohn)

Urinary system

1. Urinary tract infection or UTI (infección de vías urinarias or IVU)

2. Kidney stones (cálculos renales)

3. Urinary incontinence (incontinencia urinaria)

4. Chronic kidney disease or CKD (enfermedad renal crónica or ERC)

5. Bladder cancer (cáncer de vejiga)

6. Pyelonephritis (pielonefritis)

7. Interstitial cystitis (cistitis intersticial)

8. Benign prostatic hyperplasia (hiperplasia prostática benigna)

9. Glomerulonephritis (glomerulonefritis)

10. Nephrotic syndrome (síndrome nefrótico)

Musculoskeletal system

1. Osteoarthritis (osteoartritis)

2. Rheumatoid arthritis (artritis reumatoide)

3. Fractures (fracturas)

4. Sprains (esguinces)

5. Herniated disc (hernia de disco or hernia discal)

6. Gout (gota)

7. Carpal tunnel syndrome (syndrome del túnel del carpo)

8. Osteoporosis (osteoporosis)

9. Tendinitis (tendinitis)

10. Bursitis (bursitis)

Nervous system

1. Alzheimer's disease (enfermedad de Alzheimer)

2. Parkinson's disease (enfermedad de Parkinson)

3. Epilepsy (epilepsia)

4. Dementia (demencia)

5. Stroke (accidente cerebrovascular or ACV)

6. Concussion (concusión)

7. Multiple sclerosis (esclerosis múltiple)

8. Amyotrophic lateral sclerosis or ALS (esclerosis lateral amiotrófica or ELA)

9. Migraine (migraña)

10. Cerebral palsy (parálisis cerebral)

Visual system

1. Cataract (catarata)

2. Glaucoma (glaucoma)

3. Diabetic retinopathy (retinopatía diabética)

4. Conjunctivitis (conjuntivitis)

5. Strabismus (estrabismo)

6. Macular degeneration (degeneración macular)

7. Astigmatism (astigmatismo)

8. Myopia (miopía)

9. Hyperopia (hipermetropía)

10. Presbyopia (presbicia)

Examples of conversations between doctor/nurses and patients

Below, you will find sample conversations between healthcare professionals and patients, designed to help you practice using the anatomy and physiology terms, medical conditions and diseases, and vocabulary you have learned in this chapter.

Conversation 1: Musculoskeletal system

	Spanish		English
Doctor	Hola, ¿cómo se siente hoy?	Doctor	Hello, how are you feeling today?
Paciente	Hola, doctor. Me duele la rodilla derecha.	Patient	Hi, doctor. My right knee hurts.
Doctor	¿Desde cuándo le duele?	Doctor	For how long has it been hurting?
Paciente	Desde hace unos días.	Patient	For a few days.
Doctor	Debe ser algo relacionado a los músculos o los huesos. ¿Ha tenido algún golpe o caída reciente?	Doctor	It must be something related to the bone or muscle. Have you had any recent hits or falls?
Paciente	No, no que yo recuerde.	Patient	No, not that I remember.

	Spanish		English
Doctor	Entonces, puede ser una lesión en el cartílago o el tendón. Primero haré una revisión manual de sus rodillas y luego vamos a programar una radiografía y una resonancia magnética para obtener una imagen más clara. Por favor, firme el consentimiento informado para realizar los estudios y dígame si tiene alguna duda.	Doctor	Then it could be an injury to the cartilage or tendon. First, I will do a manual examination of your knees, and then we will schedule an X-ray and an MRI to get a clearer image. Please, sign the informed consent form to proceed with the tests, and let me know if you have any questions.
Paciente	De acuerdo, doctor. ¿Qué debo hacer mientras tanto?	Patient	: Okay, doctor. What should I do in the meantime?
Doctor	Le recetaré analgésicos para aliviar el dolor y le recomiendo que evite hacer ejercicio o actividades físicas que puedan empeorar el dolor.	Doctor	I will prescribe some pain killers to alleviate the pain and I recommend that you avoid exercising or engaging in physical activities that could worsen the pain.

Conversation 2: Respiratory system

	Spanish		English
Doctor	Hola, ¿cómo se siente hoy?	Doctor	Hello, how are you feeling today?
Paciente	Hola, doctor. He tenido dificultad para respirar desde hace unos días.	Patient	Hi, doctor. I've been having difficulty breathing for a few days.
Doctor	Permítame examinar sus pulmones con mi estetoscopio. Parece que tiene asma. ¿Tiene algún antecedente de asma en su familia?	Doctor	Let me examine your lungs with my stethoscope. It looks like you have asthma. Do you have any family history of asthma?
Paciente	No, no que yo sepa.	Patient	No, not that I know of.
Doctor	Le recetaré un inhalador para el asma y le recomiendo que evite el humo del tabaco y otros irritantes. Si no mejora, volveremos a evaluar su caso y podemos hacer pruebas adicionales.	Doctor	I will prescribe you an inhaler for asthma and recommend that you avoid tobacco smoke and other irritants. If there is no improvement, we will reassess your case and consider additional testing.
Paciente	De acuerdo, doctor.	Patient	Okay, doctor.

Conversation 3: Urinary Tract Infection (UTI)

	Spanish		English
Doctor	Hola, ¿cómo está hoy?	Doctor	Hi, how are you today?
Paciente	Hola, no muy bien. Tengo dolor al orinar y muchas ganas de ir al baño.	Patient	Hi, not very well. I have pain when urinating and a strong urge to go to the bathroom.
Doctor	Entiendo, esas molestias podrían indicar una infección urinaria. ¿Ha tenido esto antes?	Doctor	I understand, those symptoms may indicate a urinary infection. Have you experienced this before?
Paciente	Sí, una vez hace unos años.	Patient	Yes, once a few years ago.
Doctor	Bien, vamos a hacer un examen de orina y, si es necesario, le prescribiré antibióticos para tratar la infección. Mientras tanto, asegúrese de beber mucha agua y evitar irritantes para la vejiga como la cafeína y el alcohol.	Doctor	Alright, we're going to do a urine test and if necessary, I'll prescribe antibiotics to treat the infection. In the meantime, make sure to drink plenty of water and avoid bladder irritants like caffeine and alcohol.
Paciente	De acuerdo, gracias.	Patient	Okay, thank you.
Doctor	Los resultados del examen de orina muestran que tiene una infección de las vías urinarias. Le recetaré un antibiótico que debe tomar durante los próximos cinco días. Asegúrese de seguir las indicaciones y siga bebiendo mucha agua.	Doctor	The urine test results show that you have a urinary tract infection. I'll prescribe an antibiotic for you to take for the next five days. Make sure to follow the recommendations and continue drinking plenty of water.
Paciente	De acuerdo, lo haré. ¿Hay algo más que pueda hacer para prevenir futuras infecciones de las vías urinaria?	Patient	Alright, I will. Is there anything else I can do to prevent future urinary tract infections?
Doctor	Sí, asegúrese de orinar después de tener relaciones sexuales y siempre limpiarse de adelante hacia atrás después de ir al baño para evitar la propagación de bacterias desde el ano hacia la uretra.	Doctor	Yes, make sure to urinate after sexual intercourse and always wipe from front to back after using the bathroom to avoid the spread of bacteria from the anus to the urethra.
Paciente	Gracias, tomaré nota de eso.	Patient	Thank you, I'll take note of that.
Paciente	Gracias, tomaré nota de eso.	Patient	Thank you, I'll take note of that.

Conversation 4: Rheumatoid arthritis

	Spanish		English
Doctor	Hola, ¿cómo ha estado desde la última vez que nos vimos?	Doctor	Hi, how have you been since the last time we saw each other?
Paciente	No muy bien, tengo mucho dolor en las articulaciones y me cuesta moverme.	Patient	Not very well, I have a lot of joint pain, and it's hard for me to move.
Doctor	Entiendo. Según lo que me ha comentado, parece que podría estar experimentando inflamación en las articulaciones. Vamos a realizar algunas pruebas para confirmar el diagnóstico. ¿Está de acuerdo en hacerse estas pruebas?	Doctor	I understand. Based on what you've told me, it seems you might be experiencing joint inflammation. We will conduct some tests to confirm the diagnosis. Do you agree to undergo these tests?
Paciente	De acuerdo, espero que pueda ayudarme a sentirme mejor.	Patient	Okay, I hope you can help me feel better.
Doctor	Los resultados de las pruebas confirman que tiene artritis reumatoide, una enfermedad del sistema inmune que causa inflamación en las articulaciones. Podemos explorar varias opciones de tratamiento, como medicamentos antiinflamatorios y terapia física. La terapia física incluye ejercicios para mantener la movilidad y fortalecer los músculos alrededor de las articulaciones. Además, hacer más ejercicio y seguir una dieta saludable pueden ser útiles para mejorar su calidad de vida.	Doctor	The test results confirm that you have rheumatoid arthritis, an immune system disease that causes joint inflammation. We can explore several treatment options, such as anti-inflammatory medications and physical therapy. Physical therapy includes exercises to maintain mobility and strengthen the muscles around the joints. Additionally, exercising more and following a healthy diet can help improve your quality of life.
Paciente	¿Puedo seguir trabajando mientras estoy en tratamiento?	Patient	Can I continue working while I'm undergoing treatment?
Doctor	Depende de su trabajo y de la gravedad de su malestar. Es posible que debamos hacer algunos ajustes a su horario o tareas para que pueda manejar mejor el dolor.	Doctor	It depends on your job and the severity of your discomfort. We may need to make some adjustments to your schedule or tasks so that you can better manage the pain.
Paciente	Entiendo, gracias por su ayuda.	Patient	I understand, thank you for your help.

Key takeaways:

- Mastering basic anatomy and physiology terms are essential to communicate effectively in a medical setting.

- Understanding the parts of the body and their functions is crucial to comprehending and diagnosing medical conditions and diseases.

- Healthcare professionals must communicate with their patients in their language to provide the best possible care.

- Establishing trust and delivering accurate diagnoses and treatments require active listening and clear communication.

- The Spanish language is rich in medical vocabulary and expressions that can help healthcare professionals communicate more effectively with Spanish-speaking patients.

Exercises

Exercise 1

Translate the following medical conditions and diseases from English to Spanish.

No.	English	Spanish
1	Asthma	
2	Diabetes	
3	Arthritis	
4	High blood pressure	
5	Migraine	
6	Osteoporosis	
7	Stroke	
8	Breast cancer	
9	Prostate cancer	
10	Alzheimer's disease	

Exercise 2

Match the medical terms in Spanish with their English translations.

English	Spanish
1. Corazón	a. Liver

English	Spanish
2. Hígado	b. Brain
3. Estómago	c. Heart
4. Cerebro	d. Stomach
5.Riñón	e. Kidney

Exercise 3

Translate the following medical phrases from English to Spanish.

No.	English	Spanish
1	Can you describe your symptoms?	
2	How long have you been feeling this way?	
3	Have you been taking any medication for this?	
4	Please lie down on the examination table.	
5	Take a deep breath and hold it.	

Exercise 4

Create a dialogue between a doctor and a patient. Use at least five body parts and medical terms in Spanish.

Exercise 5

Choose the appropriate medical condition to match the given symptoms.

No.	Symptoms	Medical condition in Spanish
1	A patient complains of chest pain and difficulty breathing.	
2	A patient experiences frequent urination and increased thirst.	
3	A patient has joint pain and stiffness.	
4	A patient has a persistent cough and wheezing.	
5	A patient has sudden weakness or numbness on one side of the body.	

Answer key

Exercise 1

No.	English	Spanish
1	Asthma	Asma
2	Diabetes	Diabetes
3	Arthritis	Artritis
4	High blood pressure	Hipertensión arterial
5	Migraine	Migraña
6	Osteoporosis	Osteoporosis
7	Stroke	Accidente cerebrovascular
8	Breast cancer	Cáncer de mama
9	Prostate cancer	Cáncer de próstata
10	Alzheimer's disease	Enfermedad de Alzheimer

Exercise 2

1. c

2. a

3. d

4. b

5. e

Exercise 3

Translate the following medical phrases from English to Spanish.

No.	English	Spanish
1	Can you describe your symptoms?	¿Puede describir sus síntomas?
2	How long have you been feeling this way?	¿Cuánto tiempo ha estado sintiéndose así?
3	Have you been taking any medication for this?	¿Ha estado tomando algún medicamento para esto?
4	Please lie down on the examination table.	Por favor, acuéstese en la mesa de examen.
5	Take a deep breath and hold it.	Respire profundo y manténgalo.

Exercise 4

Dialogue example:

	Spanish		English
Doctor	Buenos días, ¿cómo se encuentra hoy?	Doctor	Good morning, how are you feeling today?
Paciente	Hola, doctor. Me duele la cabeza y tengo náuseas.	Patient	Hello, doctor. I have a headache and I feel nauseous.
Doctor	Entiendo. ¿También tiene dolor en el estómago o en el abdomen?	Doctor	I understand. Do you also have pain in your stomach or abdomen?
Paciente	Sí, me duele el estómago y he estado vomitando.	Patient	Yes, I have stomach pain, and I've been vomiting.
Doctor	De acuerdo, parece que tiene una gastroenteritis. Le recetaré unos medicamentos para aliviar el dolor abdominal y las náuseas. También le sugiero que beba mucho líquido y descanse lo suficiente para que su cuerpo pueda recuperarse.	Doctor	Alright, it seems you have gastroenteritis. I will prescribe some medication to relieve your abdominal pain and nausea. I also suggest you drink plenty of fluids and get enough rest so your body can recover.
Paciente	Doctor, también tengo dolor en la espalda y en el cuello.	Patient	Doctor, I also have pain in my back and neck.
Doctor	Esto puede ser debido a la tensión muscular. Le recetaré unos relajantes musculares para aliviar el dolor. Además, asegúrese de mantener una buena postura mientras está sentado o de pie para evitar la tensión muscular en el futuro.	Doctor	This could be due to muscle tension. I will prescribe some muscle relaxants to relieve the pain. Additionally, make sure to maintain good posture while sitting or standing to avoid muscle tension in the future.
Paciente	Muchas gracias, doctor.	Patient	Thank you very much, doctor.

Exercise 5

Choose the appropriate medical condition to match the given symptoms.

No.	Symptoms	Medical condition in Spanish
1	A patient complains of chest pain and difficulty breathing.	Infarto al miocardio

No.	Symptoms	Medical condition in Spanish
2	A patient experiences frequent urination and increased thirst.	Diabetes
3	A patient has joint pain and stiffness.	Artritis
4	A patient has a persistent cough and wheezing.	Asma
5	A patient has sudden weakness or numbness on one side of the body.	Accidente cerebrovascular

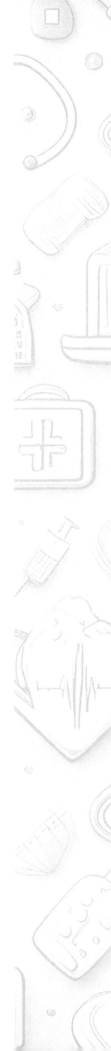

Chapter 2:
Medical Procedures and Exams

La agonía física, biológica, natural, de un cuerpo por hambre, sed o frío, dura poco, muy poco, pero la agonía del alma insatisfecha dura toda la vida.

Federico García Lorca

This chapter explores essential medical vocabulary, common questions and phrases, patient instructions, and conversational examples. Mastering this content empowers healthcare professionals to create positive interactions with Spanish-speaking patients and ensure comprehensive, high-quality treatment.

We will begin by introducing key medical terminology, including terms like "prueba de sangre" (blood test), "radiografía de tórax" (chest x-ray), "resonancia magnética" (MRI), and more. Next, we will provide common questions and phrases to help healthcare professionals establish connections with patients and understand their medical history and symptoms. Also, we will offer instructions to help healthcare professionals communicate effectively with their patients during and after medical procedures and examinations.

Vocabulary for medical procedures and exams in Spanish

Spanish	English
Tomografía computarizada or TAC	Computed tomography or CT scan
Radiografía or RX	X-ray
Resonancia magnética or RM	Magnetic Resonance Imaging or MRI
Electrocardiograma or ECG	Electrocardiogram or ECG
Examen de sangre	Blood tests

Spanish	English
Examen general de orina, urianálisis or EGO	Urine test, urinalysis
Examen de heces	Stool test
Endoscopía	Endoscopy
Colonoscopía	Colonoscopy
Biopsia	Biopsy
Cirugía	Surgery
Anestesia	Anesthesia
Terapia física	Physical therapy
Terapia ocupacional	Occupational therapy
Terapia del habla	Speech therapy
Terapia respiratoria	Respiratory therapy
Hemodiálisis	Hemodialysis
Quimioterapia	Chemotherapy
Radioterapia	Radiation therapy
Trasplante	Transplant
Paraclínico	Paraclinical

Common questions and phrases during patient consultations

Asking questions and using phrases in medical Spanish can help patients feel more comfortable and improve communication. Here are some commonly used questions and phrases that can be useful during patient consultations:

Questions:

Spanish	English
¿Qué síntomas tiene?	What symptoms do you have?
¿Cuál es su malestar/ dolencia/ condición?	What is your discomfort/ailment/condition?
¿Desde cuándo ha tenido estos síntomas?	How long have you had these symptoms?
¿Ha tenido esto antes?	Have you had this before?

Spanish	English
¿Está tomando algún medicamento actualmente?	Are you currently taking any medication?
¿Tiene alguna alergia a algún medicamento?	Do you have any allergies to medication?
¿Ha tenido alguna cirugía antes?	Have you had any surgery before?
¿Ha tenido alguna enfermedad importante en el pasado?	Have you had any significant illness in the past?
¿Tiene algún problema médico crónico?	Do you have any chronic medical condition?
¿Ha estado en contacto con alguien que tenga COVID-19?	Have you been in contact with someone who has COVID-19?
¿Está vacunado contra COVID-19?	Are you vaccinated against COVID-19?
¿Alguien más en su casa o en el trabajo tiene estos síntomas?	Does anyone else at your home or work have these symptoms?
¿Cuántas veces al día está tomando este medicamento?	How many times a day are you taking this medication?
¿Cuándo fue la última vez que se hizo exámenes de laboratorio?	When was the last time you had lab tests done?
¿En su familia hay antecedentes de esta enfermedad?	Is there a family history of this disease?

Phrases:

Spanish	English
Hablemos sobre su historial médico.	Let's talk about your medical history.
Vamos a realizar algunos exámenes para diagnosticar su problema.	We will perform some tests to diagnose your problem.
¿Usted estaría de acuerdo en realizarse estos exámenes?	Would you agree to undergo these tests?
¿Me permite examinarlo?	May I examine you?
Por favor, siéntese aquí.	Please, have a seat here.
Por favor, respire profundo.	Please, take a deep breath.
No se preocupe, estamos aquí para ayudarlo.	Don't worry, we are here to help you.
Es posible que sienta un poco de molestia.	You may feel some discomfort.
Necesito que se descubra el pecho.	I need you to uncover your chest.

Spanish	English
Por favor, espere aquí	Please, wait here.
Necesitamos que regrese para más exámenes.	We need you to come back for more tests-
Necesito palpar esta zona como parte del examen físico.	I need to palpate this area as part of the physical exam.

How to give instructions to patients in Spanish

Clear instructions in medical Spanish help patients understand their required actions. Here are some examples of effective patient instruction techniques:

Spanish	English
Tomar la medicación dos veces al día después de las comidas.	Take the medication twice a day after meals.
Beber mucha agua antes del ultrasonido pélvico.	Drink plenty of water before the pelvic ultrasound.
No comer nada después de la medianoche antes de la cirugía.	Do not eat anything after midnight before surgery.
Mantener el área limpia y seca después de la cirugía.	Keep the area clean and dry after surgery.
Descansar y evitar actividades físicas pesadas después de la cirugía.	Rest and avoid heavy physical activities after surgery.
Usar la silla de ruedas si tiene dificultades para caminar.	Use the wheelchair if you have difficulty walking.
Cambiar el vendaje y aplicar la crema en la herida según las instrucciones.	Change the bandage and apply the cream to the wound as directed
Hacer ejercicios de terapia física según lo indicado.	Do physical therapy exercises as directed.
Evitar comer alimentos grasosos y picantes después de la endoscopia.	Avoid eating fatty and spicy foods after endoscopy.
No tomar nada por vía oral después de la medianoche antes de la colonoscopia.	Do not take anything orally after midnight before the colonoscopy.
Realizar ejercicios de respiración profunda después de la cirugía del pecho.	Perform deep breathing exercises after chest surgery.
Usar la máscara de oxígeno según lo indicado.	Use the oxygen mask as directed.
Aplicar hielo en la zona lesionada para reducir la hinchazón.	Apply ice to the injured area to reduce swelling.

Spanish	English
Usar un protector solar con un alto factor de protección después de la terapia de radiación.	Use a high-SPF sunscreen after radiation therapy.
Evitar conducir después de recibir anestesia.	Avoid driving after receiving anesthesia.

Examples of conversations between doctors/nurses and patients

Conversation 1:

	Spanish		English
Doctor	Hola, ¿cómo está hoy?	Doctor	Hi, how are you feeling today?
Paciente	Estoy bien, gracias.	Patient	I'm fine, thank you.
Doctor	Dígame, ¿cuál es el problema?	Doctor	Tell me, what is the problem?
Paciente	Tengo dolor de cabeza y fiebre.	Patient	I have a headache and a fever.
Doctor	¿Desde cuándo ha tenido estos síntomas?	Doctor	How long have you had these symptoms?
Paciente	Desde ayer por la noche.	Patient	Since last night.
Doctor	¿Alguien más en su casa o trabajo tiene síntomas similares?	Doctor	Does anyone else at your home or work have similar symptoms?
Paciente	No, doctor.	Patient	No, doctor.
Doctor	Bien, vamos a realizar algunos exámenes para ver qué está causando su dolor de cabeza y fiebre. También le daré medicamentos para reducir su dolor y fiebre. ¿Tiene alguna alergia a algún medicamento?	Doctor	Alright, we're going to run some tests to see what's causing your headache and fever. I'll also give you medication to help reduce your pain and fever. Do you have any allergies to any medication?
Paciente	Sí, soy alérgico a la penicilina.	Patient	Yes, I'm allergic to penicillin.
Doctor	Muy bien, tendremos en cuenta su alergia al elegir su medicina. ¿Tiene alguna otra pregunta o preocupación?	Doctor	Okay, we'll take note of your allergy when choosing your medication. Do you have any other questions or concerns?
Paciente	No, eso es todo. Gracias, doctor.	Patient	No, that's all. Thank you, doctor

Conversation 2:

	Spanish		English
Enfermero	Hola, soy el enfermero que lo va a preparar para su cirugía. ¿Está listo para que empecemos?	Nurse	Hello, I'm the nurse who will be preparing you for your surgery. Are you ready to begin?
Paciente	Sí, estoy listo.	Patient	Yes, I'm ready.

	Spanish		English
Enfermero	Antes de la cirugía, necesitará quitarse toda la ropa y ponerse esta bata de hospital. También necesitará quitarse cualquier joya o prótesis dental. ¿Tiene alguna pregunta?	Nurse	Before the surgery, you'll need to remove all your clothing and put on this hospital gown. You'll also need to remove any jewelry or dental prostheses. Do you have any questions?
Paciente	No, eso está bien.	Patient	No, that's okay.
Enfermero	Bien, ahora vamos a ponerle una vía intravenosa para administrarle los medicamentos durante la cirugía. También le daremos algunos medicamentos para ayudarlo a relajarse antes de la cirugía. ¿Tiene alguna pregunta o preocupación?	Nurse	Okay, now we're going to insert an intravenous line to administer medications during the surgery. We'll also give you some medication to help you relax before the surgery. Do you have any questions or concerns?
Paciente	No, estoy un poco nervioso, pero confío en que todo saldrá bien.	Patient	No, I'm a little nervous, but I trust everything will go well.
Enfermero	No se preocupe, estará en buenas manos. Vamos a prepararlo para la cirugía ahora.	Nurse	Don't worry, you'll be in good hands. Let's prepare you for the surgery now.

Conversation 3:

	Spanish		English
Doctor	Hola, ¿cómo ha estado desde su última visita?	Doctor	Hello, how have you been since your last visit?
Paciente	He estado bien, gracias.	Patient	I've been good, thank you.
Doctor:	Hoy vamos a realizar una endoscopia para ver si hay algún problema en su estómago. ¿Ha seguido las indicaciones para prepararse para la prueba?	Doctor	Today we're going to perform an endoscopy to see if there's any problem in your stomach. Have you followed the instructions to prepare for the test?

	Spanish		English
Paciente	Sí, he seguido las instrucciones y no he comido nada en las últimas 12 horas.	Patient	Yes, I have followed the instructions and haven't eaten anything in the last 12 hours.
Doctor	Muy bien, eso es importante para que podamos obtener una imagen clara de su estómago. Durante la prueba, le daremos un sedante para que se sienta más cómodo. ¿Tiene alguna pregunta o preocupación?	Doctor	Very good, that's important so we can get a clear image of your stomach. During the test, we'll give you a sedative to make you more comfortable. Do you have any questions or concerns?
Paciente	¿Cómo será la prueba?	Patient	What will the test be like?
Doctor	Insertaremos un tubo flexible en su boca y lo guiaremos hacia su estómago para verlo con una cámara. No sentirá dolor, pero puede sentir algo de presión. La prueba suele durar unos 30 minutos. ¿Tiene alguna otra pregunta?	Doctor	We'll insert a flexible tube through your mouth and guide it down to your stomach to see it with a camera. You won't feel any pain, but you may feel some pressure. The test usually lasts about 30 minutes. Do you have any other questions?
Paciente	No, está bien. Gracias, doctor.	Patient	No, it's okay. Thank you, doctor.

Conversation 4:

	Spanish		English
Enfermera	Hola, soy la enfermera encargada de su cuidado después de la cirugía. ¿Cómo se siente?	Nurse	Hi, I'm the nurse in charge of your care after surgery. How are you feeling?
Paciente	Me duele mucho el área donde me operaron.	Patient	The area where I was operated on hurts a lot.
Enfermera	Eso es normal después de la cirugía. Le daremos medicamentos para el dolor. ¿Ha estado respirando profundamente como le indicamos?	Nurse	That's normal after surgery. We will give you pain medication. Have you been taking deep breaths as instructed?
Paciente	Sí, he estado haciendo los ejercicios de respiración.	Patient	Yes, I have been doing the breathing exercises.

	Spanish		English
Enfermera	Muy bien, eso es importante para prevenir complicaciones después de la cirugía. También necesitamos que se mueva un poco para prevenir coágulos de sangre. ¿Puede levantarse y caminar un poco con nuestra ayuda?	Nurse	Very good, that's important to prevent complications after surgery. We also need you to move a little to prevent blood clots. Can you try to get up and walk a bit with our help?
Paciente	Sí, puedo intentarlo.	Patient	Yes, I can try.
Enfermera	Muy bien, vamos a ayudarlo a levantarse y caminar. ¿Tiene alguna otra pregunta o preocupación?	Nurse	Great, we'll help you get up and walk. Do you have any other questions or concerns?
Paciente	No, eso es todo por ahora. Gracias, enfermera.	Patient	No, that's all for now. Thank you, nurse.

Key takeaways

- Acquiring medical Spanish vocabulary for procedures and exams is essential for healthcare professionals working with Spanish-speaking patients.

- Employing common questions and phrases for patient consultations can help establish clear communication with patients.

- Providing instructions to patients in Spanish requires clear and concise language to ensure they understand what they need to do.

- Effective communication in healthcare professional-patient interactions varies with each situation, fostering understanding and building rapport.

Exercises

Exercise 1

Translate the following medical procedures into Spanish:

No.	English	Spanish
1	Blood test	
2	Chest X-ray	
3	MRI	
4	Physical therapy	
5	Endoscopy	

Exercise 2

Complete the following sentences with the correct vocabulary:

a. Después de la cirugía, es importante mantener el área _____ y _____.

b. La endoscopia es un procedimiento para examinar el _____.

c. La _____ es un tipo de terapia que ayuda a mejorar la movilidad

d. La _____ se utiliza para obtener imágenes detalladas del cuerpo.

e. Durante la radiografía de tórax, el paciente debe _____.

Exercise 3

Match the following questions with their appropriate answers:

a. ¿Cómo se siente?

b. ¿Ha seguido las indicaciones?

c. ¿Qué le duele?

d. ¿Cuánto tiempo durará la prueba?

e. ¿Qué vamos a hacer hoy?

i. Vamos a realizar una endoscopia para ver si hay algún problema en su estómago.

ii. Me duele mucho el área donde me operaron.

iii. Me siento mareado.

iv. La prueba suele durar unos 30 minutos.

v. Sí, he seguido las instrucciones y no he comido nada en las últimas 12 horas.

Exercise 4

Write instructions in Spanish for the following situations:

No.	English	Spanish
1	Instruct a patient to take their medication twice a day with food.	
2	Instruct a patient to drink plenty of water before their MRI.	
3	Instruct a patient to avoid eating or drinking anything after midnight before their surgery.	

Exercise 5

Write a conversation between a doctor and a patient about the patient's upcoming surgery. Use at least 10 vocabulary words related to medical procedures and exams.

Answer key

Exercise 1

No.	English	Spanish
1	Blood test	Prueba de sangre
2	Chest X-ray	Radiografía de tórax
3	MRI	Resonancia magnética (RM)
4	Physical therapy	Terapia física
5	Endoscopy	Endoscopía

Exercise 2

a. Después de la cirugía, es importante mantener el área limpia y **seca**.

b. La endoscopia es un procedimiento para examinar el **estómago**.

c. La **terapia física** es un tipo de terapia que ayuda a mejorar la movilidad

d. La **resonancia magnética** utiliza para obtener imágenes detalladas del cuerpo.

e. Durante la radiografía de tórax, el paciente debe **respirar profundamente**.

Exercise 3

a-iii, b-v, c-ii, d-iv, e-i

Exercise 4

No.	English	Spanish
1	Instruct a patient to take their medication twice a day with food.	Tome su medicamento dos veces al día con comida.
2	Instruct a patient to drink plenty of water before their MRI.	Beba mucha agua antes de su resonancia magnética.
3	Instruct a patient to avoid eating or drinking anything after midnight before their surgery.	Evite comer o beber cualquier cosa después de medianoche antes de su cirugía.

Exercise 5

Example of possible dialogue:

Spanish		English	
Doctor	Hola, ¿cómo se siente hoy?	Doctor	Hello, how are you feeling today?
Paciente	Un poco nervioso por mi cirugía.	Patient	A bit nervous about my surgery.

	Spanish		English
Doctor	No se preocupe, todo saldrá bien. ¿Ha seguido las indicaciones antes de la cirugía?	Doctor	Don't worry, everything will be fine. Have you followed the pre-surgery instructions?
Paciente	Sí, he dejado de comer y beber desde la noche anterior.	Patient	Yes, I stopped eating and drinking since the night before.
Doctor	Perfecto. Durante la cirugía, le administraremos anestesia para que no sienta dolor. También le pondremos una vía intravenosa para administrarle medicamentos durante la cirugía. Después de la cirugía, necesitará descansar y recuperarse. ¿Tiene alguna otra pregunta?	Doctor	Perfect. During the surgery, we will administer anesthesia, so you won't feel any pain. We will also place an intravenous line to give you medication during the surgery. After the surgery, you will need to rest and recover. Do you have any other questions?
Paciente	¿Cuánto tiempo durará la cirugía?	Patient	How long will the surgery last?
Doctor	La cirugía debería durar unas dos horas. Estaremos monitoreando su condición durante todo el procedimiento. ¿Tiene alguna otra pregunta o preocupación?	Doctor	The surgery should last about two hours. We will be monitoring your condition throughout the procedure. Do you have any other questions or concerns?
Paciente	No, eso es todo. Gracias, doctor.	Patient	No, that's all. Thank you, doctor.

Chapter 3:
Prescription and Medication

El buen médico trata la enfermedad; el gran médico trata al paciente que tiene la enfermedad.

William Osler

In this chapter, we will delve into the essential Spanish vocabulary and phrases related to prescription and medication. Understanding and administering medications correctly impact patient well-being in healthcare settings. By the end of this chapter, you will learn:

- Identify Spanish terms for prescription and medication.

- Inquire about allergies and side effects in Spanish.

- Explain dosage and instructions in Spanish.

- List common prescription (R.X.) and over-the-counter (OTC) medications in Spanish.

- Provide examples of conversations between doctors/nurses and patients.

Spanish terms for prescriptions and medications

In Spanish, "receta médica," refers to a prescription, while "medicamento" denotes medication. Prescriptions are typically issued by a doctor ("médico") or a nurse practitioner ("enfermero(a) practicante"). Below are ten essential terms related to prescriptions and medications in Spanish:

Spanish	English
Antibiótico	Antibiotic
Antiinflamatorio	Anti-inflammatory
Analgésico	Analgesic

Spanish	English
Antihipertensivos	Antihypertensives
Insulina	Insulin
Esteroides	Steroids
Vacuna	Vaccine
Antidepresivo	Antidepressant

How to inquire about allergies and side effects in Spanish

Inquiring about allergies and potential side effects of medications ensures the safety and well-being of your patient. Ask these questions with confidence and accuracy to avoid any adverse reactions and deliver proper care. Below are ten comprehensive examples of questions in Spanish related to allergies and side effects, along with their English translations:

Spanish	English
¿Es alérgico a algún medicamento?	Are you allergic to any medication?
¿Ha tenido alguna reacción alérgica a algún medicamento en el pasado?	Have you ever had an allergic reaction to any medication in the past?
¿Ha experimentado algún efecto secundario con este medicamento?	Have you experienced any side effects with this medication?
¿Tiene alergia a algún alimento en específico o algún otro componente?	Do you have an allergy to any specific food or any other ingredient?
¿Le han recetado este medicamento anteriormente?	Have you been prescribed this medication before?
¿Hay algún medicamento que no pueda tomar?	Is there any medication you cannot take?
¿Experimentó náuseas, vómitos o mareos con este medicamento?	Did you experience nausea, vomiting, or dizziness with this medication?
¿Siente algún dolor o molestia después de tomar el medicamento?	Do you feel any pain or discomfort after taking the medication?
¿Ha notado alguna mejora desde que comenzó a tomar este medicamento?	Have you noticed any improvement since you started taking this medication?
¿Es usted alérgico a los antiinflamatorios no esteroideos (AINEs)?	Are you allergic to non-steroidal anti-inflammatory drugs (NSAIDs)?

How to explain dosage and instructions in Spanish

Appropriately conveying dosage and instructions for medication ensures that patients adhere accurately and safely to the prescribed treatment regimen. This enhances the medication's effectiveness and prevents potential side effects or complications. To assist you in providing accurate and concise information, we have compiled a list of ten essential phrases for explaining dosage and instructions in Spanish:

Spanish	English
Tome una pastilla cada ocho horas.	Take one pill every eight hours.
Tome dos pastillas al día, una por la mañana y otra por la noche.	Take two pills a day, one in the morning and one at night.
Aplique el ungüento en la zona afectada dos veces al día.	Apply the ointment to the affected area twice per day.
Use el inhalador según sea necesario, pero no más de cuatro veces al día.	Use the inhaler as needed, but no more than four times per day.
Inyecte la insulina antes de cada comida.	Inject insulin before each meal.
Agite bien el medicamento antes de usarlo.	Shake the medication well before using it.
No tome este medicamento con el estómago vacío.	Do not take this medication on an empty stomach.
Beba un vaso lleno de agua con cada dosis.	Drink a full glass of water with each dose.
No consuma alcohol mientras toma este medicamento.	Do not consume alcohol while taking this medication.
Si experimenta efectos secundarios graves, comuníquese con su médico de inmediato.	If you experience severe side effects, contact your doctor immediately.
Si experimenta efectos secundarios graves, comuníquese con su médico de inmediato.	If you experience severe side effects, contact your doctor immediately.

Common R.X. and OTC medications in Spanish

In medicine, medications fall into two primary categories: prescription medications (R.X.) and over-the-counter medications (OTC).

Prescription medications require a prescription from a licensed healthcare professional due to their potency and potential side effects. They are tailored for specific medical conditions, with dosage and treatment duration carefully prescribed by healthcare providers.

On the other hand, over-the-counter medications are available without a prescription and can be purchased directly from a pharmacy or store. These medications typically address mild to moderate symptoms such as pain, fever, allergies, and indigestion, which are generally non-serious conditions. They are considered safe when used according to recommended guidelines.

In this medical book, we will focus on the most common prescription (R.X.) and over-the-counter (OTC) medications in Spanish. This knowledge ensures patients receive appropriate medications and dosages tailored to their medical needs, while also minimizing the risk of harmful drug interactions.

Detailed below are 20 examples of common prescription and over-the-counter medications in Spanish:

R.X. medications:

Spanish	English
Amoxicilina	Amoxicillin
Cefalexina	Cephalexin
Paracetamol (acetaminofén)	Paracetamol (Acetaminophen)
Ibuprofeno	Ibuprofen
Diazepam	Diazepam
Omeprazol	Omeprazole
Enalapril	Enalapril
Metformina	Metformin
Simvastatina	Simvastatin
Insulina	Insulin
Prednisona	Prednisone
Furosemida	Furosemide
Alprazolam	Alprazolam
Ranitidina	Ranitidine
Atorvastatina	Atorvastatin
Losartán	Losartan
Amoxicilina con ácido clavulánico	Amoxicillin with Clavulanic Acid
Metoprolol	Metoprolol
Clonazepam	Clonazepam
Levotiroxina	Levothyroxine
Dexametasona	Dexamethasone
Hidrocortisona	Hydrocortisone

Spanish	English
Ceftriaxona	Ceftriaxone
Fluoxetina	Fluoxetine

OTC medications:

Spanish	English
Aspirina	Aspirin
Loratadina	Loratadine
Ranitidina	Ranitidine
Naproxeno	Naproxen
Antiácidos	Antiacids
Vitamina C	Vitamin C
Dextrometorfano	Dextromethorphan
Salbutamol	Salbutamol
Ibuprofeno con pseudoefedrina	Ibuprofen with Pseudoephedrine
Ketoprofeno	Ketoprofen
Paracetamol con pseudoefedrina	Paracetamol with Pseudoephedrine
Acetaminofén con codeína	Acetaminophen with Codeine
Clorfeniramina	Chlorpheniramine
Loperamida	Loperamide
Lansoprazol	Lansoprazole
Metamizol	Metamizole
Magnesio	Magnesium
Cetirizina	Cetirizine
Probióticos	Probiotics
Lágrimas artificiales	Lubricant eye drops

Examples of conversations between doctor/nurses and patients

Conversation 1:

	Spanish		English
Doctor	Hola, ¿cómo se siente hoy?	Doctor	Hi, how are you feeling today?
Paciente	Hola doctor, me duele mucho la garganta y tengo fiebre.	Patient	Hi doctor, my throat hurts a lot and I have a fever.
Doctor	Entiendo, ¿cuántos días lleva con estos síntomas?	Doctor	I understand, how long have you had these symptoms?
Paciente	Aproximadamente tres días.	Patient	About three days.
Doctor	¿Ha tomado algún medicamento para aliviar el dolor o la fiebre?	Doctor	Have you taken any medication to relieve the pain or fever?
Paciente	Solo he tomado paracetamol, pero no me ha ayudado mucho.	Patient	I've only taken paracetamol, but it hasn't helped much.
Doctor	Usaré un abatelenguas y mi linterna para revisar su garganta. Al parecer es una infección bacteriana. ¿Es alérgico a algún medicamento?	Doctor	I will use a tongue depressor and my flashlight to examine your throat. It seems to be a bacterial infection. Are you allergic to any medications?
Paciente	Sí, soy alérgico a la penicilina.	Patient	Yes, I'm allergic to penicillin.
Doctor	De acuerdo, le recetaré un antibiótico diferente llamado azitromicina. Tome una tableta al día durante cinco días. También puede seguir tomando paracetamol para aliviar el dolor y la fiebre.	Doctor	Alright, I'll prescribe a different antibiotic called azithromycin. Take one tablet a day for five days. You can also continue taking paracetamol to relieve the pain and fever.
Paciente	¿Este medicamento puede provocarme algún otro efecto que deba tener en cuenta?	Patient	Can this medication cause any other effects that I should be aware of?

	Spanish		English
Doctor	Los efectos secundarios más comunes de la azitromicina incluyen náuseas, vómitos, diarrea y dolor de estómago. Si experimenta algún efecto secundario grave, como dificultad para respirar o erupción cutánea, comuníquese con nuestra oficina de inmediato.	Doctor	The most common side effects of azithromycin include nausea, vomiting, diarrhea, and stomach pain. If you experience any severe side effects, such as difficulty breathing or a rash, please contact our office immediately.
Paciente	Entiendo. Gracias, doctor.	Patient	I understand. Thank you, doctor.

Conversation 2:

	Spanish		English
Enfermera	Buenos días, ¿cómo puedo ayudarle hoy?	Nurse	Good morning, how can I assist you today?
Paciente	Hola, estoy aquí para recoger mi receta para la insulina.	Patient	Hi, I'm here to pick up my prescription for insulin.
Enfermera	De acuerdo, permítame verificar su información. Mientras tanto, ¿tiene alguna pregunta sobre cómo administrar la insulina?	Nurse	Alright, let me check your information. In the meantime, do you have any questions about how to administer insulin?
Paciente	Sí, ¿puede recordarme cuántas unidades debo inyectar antes de las comidas?	Patient	Yes, can you remind me how many units I should inject before meals?
Enfermera	Claro, según la receta de su médico, debe inyectarse 10 unidades de insulina antes de cada comida. Asegúrese de seguir las instrucciones al pie de la letra.	Nurse	Sure, according to your doctor's prescription, you should inject 10 units of insulin before each meal. Make sure to follow the instructions carefully.
Paciente	También tengo una pregunta sobre cómo almacenar la insulina.	Patient	I also have a question about how to store insulin.
Enfermera	Guarde la insulina en el refrigerador hasta que esté lista para usarla. Una vez que la empiece a utilizar, puede guardarla a temperatura ambiente durante un máximo de 28 días. Recuerde no exponerla a temperaturas extremas o luz solar directa.	Nurse	Store the insulin in the refrigerator until you are ready to use it. Once you start using it, you can store it at room temperature for a maximum of 28 days. Remember not to expose it to extreme temperatures or direct sunlight.

	Spanish		English
Paciente	Gracias por la información.	Patien	Thank you for the information.

Conversation 3:

	Spanish		English
Doctor	Hola, ¿cómo ha estado desde nuestra última cita?	Doctor	Hi, how have you been since our last appointment?
Paciente	Hola doctor, he estado siguiendo las recomendaciones para la presión arterial, pero todavía no veo mucha mejoría.	Patient	Hi doctor, I have been following the recommendations for my blood pressure, but I still don't see much improvement.
Doctor	¿Ha estado tomando el medicamento para la presión arterial según las indicaciones?	Doctor	Have you been taking the blood pressure medication as instructed?
Paciente	Sí, tomo una pastilla de losartán todos los días por la mañana.	Patient	Yes, I take one losartan pill every morning.
	Spanish		English
Doctor	Bien, también es importante mantener una dieta baja en sal y hacer ejercicio regularmente. ¿Ha estado haciendo cambios en su estilo de vida?	Doctor	Good. It is also important to maintain a low-salt diet and exercise regularly. Have you been making lifestyle changes?
Paciente	He intentado, pero me cuesta mantener una rutina.	Patient	I have tried, but I find it hard to maintain a routine.
Doctor	Comprendo que puede ser difícil, pero es importante para controlar su presión arterial. Podemos considerar ajustar su medicina si es necesario, pero antes, sigamos trabajando en cambios en su estilo de vida. Puedo recomendarle a un dietista y un especialista en ejercicio para ayudarle en este proceso.	Doctor	I understand that it can be difficult, but it is important for controlling your blood pressure. We can consider adjusting your medication, if necessary, but let's keep working on lifestyle changes first. I can recommend a dietitian and an exercise specialist to help you in this process.
Paciente	Eso sería de gran ayuda, gracias doctor	Patient	That would be very helpful, thank you, doctor.

Conversation 4:

	Spanish		English
Enfermera	Hola, ¿en qué puedo ayudarle hoy?	Nurse	Hello, how can I assist you today?

Spanish		English	
Paciente	Hola, mi médico me recetó un inhalador para el asma, pero no estoy seguro de cómo usarlo correctamente.	Patient	Hi, my doctor prescribed me an inhaler for asthma, but I'm not sure how to use it properly.
Enfermera	Claro, puedo mostrarle cómo hacerlo. Primero, agite el inhalador durante unos segundos. Luego, saque el aire de sus pulmones y coloque el inhalador en la boca, asegurándose de que esté bien sellado alrededor de sus labios. Presione la parte superior del inhalador para liberar la medicina mientras inhala lentamente y profundamente.	Nurse	Sure, I can show you how to do it. First, shake the inhaler for a few seconds. Then, exhale all the air from your lungs and place the inhaler in your mouth, making sure it is well sealed around your lips. Press the top of the inhaler to release the medicine while inhaling slowly and deeply.
Spanish		**English**	
Paciente	¿Cuánto tiempo debo inhalar?	Patient	How long should I inhale for?
Enfermera	Intente inhalar durante unos cinco segundos, luego sostenga la respiración durante 10 segundos para permitir que la medicina se distribuya en los pulmones. Si necesita más de una inhalación, espere al menos un minuto antes de repetir el proceso.	Nurse	Try inhaling for about five seconds, then hold your breath for 10 seconds to allow the medicine to distribute into your lungs. If you need more than one inhalation, wait at least one minute before repeating the process.
Paciente	Gracias por la explicación, ahora me siento más seguro al usar mi inhalador.	Patient	Thank you for the explanation, I now feel more confident using my inhaler.

Key takeaways

- Familiarize yourself with essential terms related to prescriptions and medications in Spanish, such as "receta médica" (prescription) and "medicamento" (medication).

- Learn to ask about allergies and side effects in Spanish to ensure patient safety and improve communication.

- Be able to explain dosage and instructions in Spanish, as proper understanding and administration of medications can greatly impact a patient's well-being.

- Know common prescription (R.X.) and over-the-counter (OTC) medications in Spanish to help patients understand their prescribed treatments.

- Practice conversation examples to improve your communication skills in real-life healthcare situations.

Exercises

Exercise 1

Match the Spanish medication name with its English translation.

Spanish	English
1.Ibuprofeno	A. Ibuprofen
2.Enalapril	B. Insulin
3.Insulina	C. Amoxicillin
4.Amoxicilina	D. Enalapril
5.Diazepam	E. Diazepam

Exercise 2

Fill in the blank with the appropriate Spanish term.

Antibióticos, medicamentos, analgésico, antihipertensivos, esteroides, vacunas, antiinflamatorios, antidepresivos.

Los _____ son utilizados para tratar la inflamación y el dolor.

Las _____ se utiliza para prevenir enfermedades infecciosas.

Los _____ se utilizan para tratar el dolor.

Los _____ son utilizados para tratar la presión arterial alta.

Los _____ se utilizan para tratar la inflamación y el dolor.

Los _____ se utilizan para tratar enfermedades mentales como la depresión.

Los _____ se utilizan para tratar infecciones bacterianas.

Los _____ se utilizan para reducir la inflamación y la hinchazón.

Exercise 3

Choose the correct Spanish term to complete the sentence.

1. ¿_____es el medicamento que está tomando?

   A. Cuál

B. Cómo

C. Dónde

D. Por qué

2. El médico me recetó un _____ para el dolor de cabeza.

A. Analgésico

B. Vitamina

C. Antibiótico

D. Vacuna

3. Tome una pastilla de _____ cada cuatro horas para la fiebre.

A. Antibiótico

B. Paracetamol

C. Antihipertensivos

D. Esteroides

4. ¿_____ algún efecto secundario con este medicamento?

A. Tiene

B. Hace

C. Come

D. Necesita

5. El _____ se aplica en la piel para tratar la inflamación.

A. Antibiótico

B. Antiinflamatorio

C. Analgésico

D. Antidepresivo

Exercise 4

Translate the following sentences into Spanish.

English	Spanish
Take one pill every eight hours.	
Apply the ointment to the affected area twice a day.	
Do not take this medication on an empty stomach.	

Exercise 5

Identify and correct the grammar mistakes in the following Spanish sentences:

Spanish sentence	Correction
Tome una pastilla cada ocha oras.	
Aplique el unguento dos veses al día.	
La vacuna no es necesario para adultos.	
El medicamento se debe tomar despuez de la comida.	
Necesito comprar un medicamento para midolor de cabeza.	

Answer key

Exercise 1

1. A
2. D
3. B
4. C
5. E

Exercise 2

Los **antiinflamatorios** son utilizados para tratar la inflamación y el dolor.

Las **vacunas** se utilizan para prevenir enfermedades infecciosas.

Los **analgésicos** se utilizan para tratar el dolor.

Los **antihipertensivos** son utilizados para tratar la presión arterial alta.

Los **esteroides** se utilizan para tratar la inflamación y el dolor.

Los **antidepresivos** se utilizan para tratar enfermedades mentales como la depresión.

Los **antibióticos** se utilizan para tratar infecciones bacterianas.

Los **antiinflamatorios** se utilizan para reducir la inflamación y la hinchazón.

Exercise 3

1. ¿_____es el medicamento que está tomando?

    A. Cuál

    B. Cómo

    C. Dónde

    D. Por qué

2. El médico me recetó un _____ para el dolor de cabeza.

    A. Analgésico

    B. Vitamina

    C. Antibiótico

    D. Vacuna

3. Tome una pastilla de _____ cada cuatro horas para la fiebre.

   A. Antibiótico

   B. Paracetamol

   C. Antihipertensivos

   D. Esteroides

4. ¿_____ algún efecto secundario con este medicamento?

   A. Tiene

   B. Hace

   C. Come

   D. Necesita

5. El _____ se aplica en la piel para tratar la inflamación.

   A. Antibiótico

   B. Antiinflamatorio

   C. Analgésico

   D. Antidepresivo

Exercise 4

English	Spanish
Take one pill every eight hours.	Tome una pastilla cada ocho horas
Apply the ointment to the affected area twice a day.	Aplique la pomada en la zona afectada dos veces al día
Do not take this medication on an empty stomach.	No tome este medicamento con el estómago vacío

Exercise 5

Identify and correct the grammar mistakes in the following Spanish sentences:

Spanish sentence	Correction
Tome una pastilla cada ocha oras.	Tome una pastilla cada ocho horas. (The correct spelling for "ocho" is with "h" meaning "eight" in English, and horas is with "h", meaning "hours" in English)

Spanish sentence	Correction
Aplique el unguento dos veses al día.	Aplique el ungüento dos veces al día. (The correct spelling is "ungüento" with "ü" meaning "ointment" in English, and "veces" instead of "veses". "Dos veces al día" means "twice a day" in English)
La vacuna no es necesario para adultos.	La vacuna no es necesaria para adultos. (The correct form is "necesaria" in feminine form, meaning "necessary" in English)
El medicamento se debe tomar despuez de la comida.	El medicamento se debe tomar después de la comida. (The correct word is "después" meaning "after" in English)
Necesito comprar un medicamento para midolor de cabeza.	This sentence is correct.

Chapter 4:
Medical Emergencies

El médico competente, antes de dar una medicina a su paciente, se familiariza no sólo con la enfermedad que desea curar, sino también con los hábitos y la constitución del enfermo.

Marco Tulio Cicerón

This chapter will focus on vocabulary and phrases for emergency situations. It will cover how to give directions to first responders, communicate with patients during an emergency, and present examples of conversations between healthcare professionals and patients. Key takeaways and interactive exercises will help you learn and practice these critical skills.

By mastering the Spanish terms presented in this chapter, you will be able to make informed decisions and respond rapidly to emergencies involving Spanish-speaking patients. Real-life examples and interactive exercises are included to reinforce your understanding of the vocabulary and phrases, enabling you to handle medical emergencies with greater competence.

Vocabulary and phrases for emergency situations

Medical emergencies can occur unexpectedly, and healthcare professionals must be prepared to provide care to patients from diverse linguistic and cultural backgrounds. Proficiency in essential Spanish vocabulary and phrases is necessary in these situations. This chapter aims to equip you with the necessary skills to navigate such scenarios confidently, allowing you to provide clear directions to first responders, communicate effectively with patients during emergencies, and understand their needs and concerns.

In an emergency, every second counts. Healthcare professionals must be able to communicate swiftly and efficiently with first responders, guiding them to the patient's location and providing crucial information about the patient's condition. This not only saves precious time but can also make a significant difference in the patient's outcome. To help you in such situations, we have compiled a list of 20 key phrases that you may need when giving directions to first responders in Spanish:

Spanish	English
Necesitamos una ambulancia en [dirección] .	We need an ambulance at [address].
Hay una emergencia en el tercer piso.	There is an emergency on the third floor.
El paciente está en la sal de espera.	The patient is in the waiting room.
Por favor, sigan a [nombre].	Please follow [name].
La entrada principal está bloqueada, usen la entrada lateral.	The main entrance is blocked, use the side entrance.
El paciente se desmayó.	The patient fainted.
La persona herida está en la esquina de [calle] y [calle].	The injured person is at the corner of [street] and [street].
El paciente no puede respirar.	The patient cannot breathe.
El paciente tiene una hemorragia.	The patient is bleeding.
El accidente de tráfico ocurrió en [ubicación].	The car accident occurred at [location].
La persona está inconsciente.	The person is unconscious.
El paciente tiene un dolor intenso en el pecho.	The patient has severe chest pain.
La persona está atrapada en el vehículo	The person is trapped in the vehicle.
Hay un incendio en [dirección].	There is a fire at [address].
El paciente tiene una reacción alérgica grave.	The patient has a severe allergic reaction.
Por favor, traigan una camilla.	Please bring a stretcher.
El paciente necesita oxígeno.	The patient needs oxygen.
La persona ha sufrido quemaduras.	The person has suffered burns.
Hay múltiples heridos.	There are multiple injured people.
El paciente está en shock.	The patient is in shock.
El paciente está convulsionando.	The patient is having a seizure.
La paciente embarazada está sangrando.	The pregnant patient is bleeding.
Estamos haciendo RCP.	We are performing CPR.
El paciente no tiene pulso.	The patient has no pulse.

How to give directions to first responders in Spanish

Effective communication during emergencies can be lifesaving, especially when dealing with language barriers. Being able to give directions to first responders in Spanish ensures timely and accurate response. This section offers 20 key phrases to help you direct first responders and provide critical information about the patient's condition in Spanish:

Spanish	English
La emergencia es en el segundo piso.	The emergency is on the second floor.
El paciente está en la sala de espera.	The patient is in the waiting room.
Por favor, diríjase a la habitación 210.	Please, go to room 210.
Hay un accidente en la entrada principal.	There is an accident at the main entrance.
Necesitamos una ambulancia en el estacionamiento.	We need an ambulance in the parking lot.
El paciente está inconsciente en el pasillo.	The patient is unconscious in the hallway.
La persona herida está al final del pasillo.	The injured person is at the end of the hallway.
Diríjase a la sala de emergencias.	Head to the emergency room.
El paciente tiene dificultad para respirar.	The patient has difficulty breathing.
Hay una situación crítica en el área de pediatría.	There is a critical situation in the pediatrics area.
Vengan al quirófano lo más rápido posible.	Come to the operating room as quickly as possible.
Necesitamos más personal en el área de trauma.	We need more staff in the trauma area.
El paciente requiere oxígeno de inmediato.	The patient requires oxygen immediately.
Trae un desfibrilador a la habitación 305.	Bring a defibrillator to room 305.
Necesitamos una camilla en el pasillo.	We need a stretcher in the hallway.
Por favor, evalúe la situación en la sala de rayos X.	Please, assess the situation in the X-ray room.
Necesitamos un médico en la sala de partos.	We need a doctor in the delivery room.
La víctima del accidente automovilístico acaba de llegar.	A car accident victim has just arrived.
Por favor, envíe a un médico a la unidad de terapia intensiva.	Please send a doctor to the intensive care unit.
Hay un incendio en el tercer piso; evacúe a los pacientes.	There is a fire on the third floor; evacuate the patients.

How to communicate with patients during an emergency in Spanish

During pressing moments, clear communication with patients can significantly impact the quality of care provided. Here are examples of phrases to use when communicating with Spanish-speaking patients in emergency situations:

Spanish	English
¿Puede respirar bien?	Can you breathe well?
¿Cuánto tiempo lleva sintiéndose así?	How long have you been feeling like this?
¿Sabe en dónde se encuentra?	Do you know where you are?
¿Perdió el conocimiento después del accidente?	Did you lose consciousness after the accident?
¿Tiene alguna alergia?	Do you have any allergies?
Voy a revisar sus signos vitales.	I'm going to check your vital signs.
¿Puede decirme su nombre completo?	Can you tell me your full name?
¿Tiene alguna enfermedad preexistente?	Do you have any pre-existing conditions?
¿Está tomando algún medicamento?	Are you taking any medication?
Vamo a llevarle al hospital.	We're going to take you to the hospital.
¿Puede mover los dedos de sus pies y manos?	Can you move your fingers and toes?
No se preocupe, está en buenas manos	Don't worry, you're in good hands
Voy a ponerle oxígeno.	I'm going to put you on oxygen.
¿Puede describir el dolor?	Can you describe the pain?
Necesito que se quedes tranquilo(a).	I need you to stay calm.
Voy a realizar una evaluación rápida.	I'm going to perform a quick assessment.
¿Ha sufrido alguna lesión en la cabeza?	Have you suffered any head injury?
¿Qué sucedió?	What happened?
¿Tiene algún familiar o amigo a quien podamos llamar?	Do you have any family or friend we can call?
Lo estamos llevando al hospital ahora mismo.	We are taking you to the hospital right now.

Mastering these phrases, along with other essential vocabulary and expressions, prepares you to effectively manage medical emergencies involving Spanish-speaking patients. This proficiency fosters trust and supports positive patient outcomes.

Examples of conversations between doctors/nurses and patients

Conversation 1:

	Spanish		English
Doctor	Buenas tardes, ¿cuál es el problema?	Doctor	Good afternoon, what is the problem?
Paciente	Comí unos camarones y ahora no puedo respirar bien. Además, me acaba de aparecer una erupción en la piel.	Patient	I ate some shrimp and now I can't breathe well. Besides, I just got a rash on my skin.
Doctor	¿Sabe si es alérgica a los camarones?	Doctor	Do you know if you are allergic to shrimp?
Paciente	No lo sé, es la primera vez que los pruebo, ayúdeme, cada vez me siento más mareada.	Patient	I don't know, this is the first time I've tried them. Help me, I'm feeling more and more dizzy.
Doctor	Permítame revisar su lengua… Parece que se está inflamanda y tiene una reacción alérgica grave. Vamos a inyectarle adrenalina, administrarle oxígeno y recostarla en una cama para observación.	Doctor	Let me check your tongue… It appears to be swollen, and you are having a severe allergic reaction. We will administer an adrenaline injection, provide you with oxygen, and place you in a bed for observation.
Paciente	Gracias, doctor.	Patient	Thank you, doctor.

Conversation 2:

	Spanish		English
Enfermera	Hola, soy la enfermera García. ¿Qué te trae al hospital?	Nurse	Hello, I am Nurse García. What brings you to the hospital?
Paciente	Me torcí el tobillo mientras jugaba fútbol.	Patient	I twisted my ankle while playing soccer.
Enfermera	¿Puede describir el dolor? ¿Es constante o intermitente?	Nurse	Can you describe the pain? Is it constant or intermittent?
Patient	Es un dolor constante y punzante.	Patient	It's a constant, sharp pain.
Enfermera	¿Ha aplicado hielo en el área lesionada?	Nurse	Have you applied ice to the injured area?

	Spanish		English
Paciente	Sí, pero el dolor sigue siendo intenso.	Patient	Yes, but the pain is still intense.
Enfermera	Vamos a revisar su tobillo y realizar algunas pruebas para determinar si hay una fractura o esguince. Mientras tanto, le proporcionaremos medicamentos para aliviar el dolor y le daremos instrucciones sobre cómo cuidar su tobillo en casa.	Nurse	We will examine your ankle and perform some tests to determine if there is a fracture or sprain. In the meantime, we will provide you with medication to relieve the pain and give you instructions on how to care for your ankle at home.
Paciente	¿Necesitaré una radiografía?	Patient	Will I need an X-ray?
Enfermera	Sí, una radiografía nos ayudará a evaluar el alcance de la lesión y a descartar cualquier fractura.	Nurse	Yes, an X-ray will help us assess the extent of the injury and rule out any fractures.
Paciente	¿Cuánto tiempo tardaré en recuperarme?	Patient	How long will it take for me to recover?
Enfermera	Dependiendo de la gravedad de la lesión, podría tardar unas pocas semanas en recuperarse completamente. Le proporcionaremos un plan de tratamiento y posiblemente le vamos a referir a un fisioterapeuta para una rehabilitación adecuada.	Nurse	Depending on the severity of the injury, it could take a few weeks to fully recover. We will provide a treatment plan and possibly refer you to a physical therapist for proper rehabilitation.

Conversation 3:

	Spanish		English
Doctor	¿Cuál es el problema?	Doctor	What is the problem?
Paciente	No puedo respirar bien y me duele el pecho.	Patient	I can't breathe well, and my chest hurts.
Doctor	¿Cuánto tiempo lleva con estos síntomas?	Doctor	How long have you had these symptoms?
Paciente	Empezaron hace unas horas.	Patient	They started a few hours ago.
Doctor	¿Tiene antecedentes de problemas cardíacos en su familia?	Doctor	Do you have a family history of heart problems?

	Spanish		English
Paciente	Sí, mi padre tuvo un infarto.	Patient	Yes, my father had a heart attack.
Doctor	Vamos a realizar un electrocardiograma y algunos análisis de sangre para evaluar su situación. Si está de acuerdo, por favor firme el consentimiento informado para proceder con estos estudios.	Doctor	We are going to perform an electrocardiogram and some blood tests to evaluate your condition. If you agree, please sign the informed consent form to proceed with these tests.
Paciente	¿Podría ser algo grave?	Patient	Could it be something serious?
Doctor	Podría serlo, pero también podrían ser síntomas de estrés o ansiedad. Es importante que estemos seguros.	Doctor	It could be, but it could also be symptoms of stress or anxiety. It's important that we are sure.
Paciente	Entiendo, ¿cuándo tendrán los resultados?	Patient	I understand, when would you have the results take?
Doctor	Los resultados del electrocardiograma estarán listos en unos minutos. Los análisis de sangre pueden tardar un poco más.	Doctor	The electrocardiogram results will be ready in a few minutes. The blood tests may take a bit longer.

Conversation 4:

	Spanish		English
Enfermera	¿Qué le sucedió?	Nurse	What happened?
Paciente	Me corté con un cuchillo mientras cocinaba.	Patient	I cut myself with a knife while I was cooking.
Enfermera	¿Sangra mucho?	Nurse	Is it bleeding a lot?
Paciente	Sí, no puedo detener el sangrado.	Patient	Yes, I can't stop the bleeding.
Enfermera	Voy a limpiar la herida y luego la suturaré.	Nurse	I will clean the wound and then suture it.
Paciente	¿Dolerá mucho?	Patient	Will it hurt a lot?
Enfermera	Aplicaremos anestesia local antes de suturar para que no sienta dolor. Pero puede sentir algo de incomodidad después.	Nurse	We will apply local anesthesia before suturing, so you won't feel pain. But you might feel some discomfort afterward.
Paciente	¿Cuánto tiempo tardará en sanar?	Patient	How long will it take to heal?

	Spanish		English
Enfermera	Depende de la profundidad de la herida y cómo la cuide. Por lo general, una herida como esta puede sanar en unas dos semanas.	Nurse	It depends on the depth of the wound and how well you care for it. Typically, a wound like this can heal in about two weeks.
Paciente	¿Hay algo que deba evitar mientras se cura?	Patient	Is there anything I should avoid while it's healing?
Enfermera	Evite mojar la herida y asegúrese de mantenerla limpia y seca. Le daré instrucciones sobre cómo cuidarla adecuadamente.	Nurse	Avoid getting the wound wet and make sure to keep it clean and dry. I will give you instructions on how to properly care for it.

Conversation 5:

	Spanish		English
Doctor	Buenas tardes ¿usted es la esposa del paciente Pérez?	Doctor	Good afternoon, are you Mr. Pérez's wife?
Acompañante	si doctor, ¿pudieron detener las convulsiones? Primera vez que le sucede algo así.	Companion	Yes, doctor. Were you able to stop the seizures? This is the first time something like this has happened to him.
Doctor	Por ahora está estable, por favor tome asiento. Le hicimos una resonancia magnética a su esposo y, por desgracia, encontramos un tumor en el cerebro.	Doctor	For now, he is stable. Please have a seat. We performed an MRI on your husband and, unfortunately, we found a tumor in his brain.
Acompañante	Dios mío, ¿cree que pueda ser cáncer?	Companion	My God, do you think it could be cancer?
Doctor	Necesitamos hacer otras pruebas y tomar una biopsia, pero es probable. En cualquier caso, haremos todo lo posible por ayudarlo.	Doctor	We need to run more tests and take a biopsy, but it is possible. In any case, we will do everything we can to help him.
Acompañante	Gracias, doctor.	Companion	Thank you, doctor.

Key takeaways

- Mastering Spanish vocabulary and phrases for effective communication with first responders and patients in emergencies enhances care for Spanish-speaking patients.

- Providing clear directions to first responders in Spanish saves time. Practice describing locations and patients' conditions for effective communication.

- Communicating with Spanish-speaking patients in emergencies involves asking about symptoms, medical history, and medications, and understanding and responding to their concerns.

- Familiarizing yourself with conversational examples between healthcare professionals and patients aids communication in emergencies.

- Regular practice of Spanish vocabulary and phrases from this chapter builds confidence in managing emergencies with Spanish-speaking patients.

Exercises

Exercise 1

Match the English phrases to their corresponding Spanish translations.

Spanish	English
Call an ambulance.	
Apply pressure to the wound.	
Perform cardiopulmonary resuscitation (CPR).	
Administer oxygen to the patient.	
Place the patient in the recovery position.	

Exercise 2

Complete the sentences with the appropriate Spanish vocabulary related to medical emergencies.

a) Necesitamos _____ médica urgente. (help)

b) _____ los signos vitales del paciente. (monitor)

c) Use un _____ para detener la hemorragia. (tourniquet)

d) Estabilice el paciente antes de _____. (transport)

e) Tenga listo el equipo de _____. (emergency)

Exercise 3

Role-playing exercise: In pairs, practice a conversation between a healthcare professional and a patient during a medical emergency. One person will act as the healthcare professional, while the other will act as the patient. Switch roles and practice the conversation again.

Exercise 4

Choose the correct Spanish translation for each English phrase.

1. Immobilize the injured area.

   Inmovilice el área lesionada.

   Inmovilice el área cortada.

   Inmovilice el área quemada.

2. Take the patient to the nearest hospital.

   Lleve al paciente al hospital más al sur.

   Lleve al paciente al hospital más lejano.

   Lleve al paciente al hospital más cercano.

3. Have the emergency equipment ready.

   Tenga lejos el equipo de urgencia.

   Tenga listo el equipo de emergencia.

   Tenga fuera el equipo de primeros auxilios.

4. Prepare the automated external defibrillator (AED).

   Prepare el desfibrilador externo automático (DEA).

   Prepare el desfibrilador automático externo (DAE).

   Prepare el desfibrilador externo automático (AED).

5. Perform cardiopulmonary resuscitation (CPR).

   Realice la resucitación cardiopulmonar (RCP).

   Realice la reanimación cardiopulmonar (RCP).

   Realice la reanimación cardiovascular (RCV).

Exercise 5

Translate the following medical emergency instructions from Spanish to English.

Spanish	English
Evacue el área	
Pida refuerzos si es necesario	
Llame al número de emergencia	
Notifique a la familia del paciente	

Answer key

Exercise 1

Spanish	English
Call an ambulance.	Llame a una ambulancia.
Apply pressure to the wound.	Aplique presión en la herida.
Perform cardiopulmonary resuscitation (CPR).	Realice la reanimación cardiopulmonar (RCP).
Administer oxygen to the patient.	Administre oxígeno al paciente.
Place the patient in the recovery position.	Coloque al paciente en posición de recuperación.

Exercise 2

Complete the sentences with the appropriate Spanish vocabulary related to medical emergencies.

a) Necesitamos **ayuda** médica urgente. (help)

b) **Monitorice** los signos vitales del paciente. (monitor)

c) Use un **torniquete** para detener la hemorragia. (tourniquet)

d) Estabilice el paciente antes de **transportarlo**. (transport)

e) Tenga listo el equipo de **emergencia**. (emergency)

Exercise 3

Example of a medical emergency conversation

Scenario: A patient has been brought to the emergency room with symptoms of a heart attack. The healthcare professional (doctor) is assessing the patient's condition and providing initial care.

	Spanish		English
Doctor	Hola, soy el Dr. López. ¿Puede decirme qué tiene?	Doctor	Hello, I'm Dr. López. Can you tell me what's wrong?
Patient	Hola, doctor. Tengo un fuerte dolor en el pecho y me falta el aire.	Patient	Hello, doctor. I have a severe chest pain and shortness of breath.
Doctor	¿Hace cuánto tiempo comenzaron las molestias?	Doctor	How long ago did the discomfort start?
Patient	Empezaron hace aproximadamente una hora.	Patient	It started about an hour ago.

	Spanish		English
Doctor	¿Ha tenido algún episodio similar antes?	Doctor	Have you had any similar episodes before?
Patient	No, esto nunca me había pasado.	Patient	No, this has never happened to me before.
Doctor	Vamos a realizar un electrocardiograma (ECG) para evaluar su corazón. Mientras tanto, voy a administrarle medicamentos para aliviar el dolor y mejorar el flujo sanguíneo. Por favor, firme el consentimiento informado si está de acuerdo.	Doctor	We are going to perform an electrocardiogram (ECG) to evaluate your heart. In the meantime, I will administer medication to relieve the pain and improve blood flow. Please sign the informed consent form if you agree.
Patient	¿Qué medicamentos me va a administrar?	Patient	What medications will you give me?
Doctor	Le daré aspirina, nitroglicerina y posiblemente un anticoagulante.	Doctor	I will give you aspirin, nitroglycerin, and possibly a blood thinner.
Patient	¿Cuál es el siguiente paso después del electrocardiograma?	Patient	What is the next step after the electrocardiogram?
Doctor	Si el ECG confirma un ataque cardíaco, podríamos realizar un cateterismo cardíaco para identificar bloqueos y tratar de abrir las arterias bloqueadas.	Doctor	If the ECG confirms a heart attack, we might perform a cardiac catheterization to identify blockages and try to open the blocked arteries.
Patient	¿Qué puedo hacer para prevenir otro ataque cardíaco en el futuro?	Patient	What can I do to prevent another heart attack in the future?
Doctor	Es importante llevar un estilo de vida saludable, que incluya una dieta equilibrada, ejercicio regular, no fumar, controlar el estrés y hacerse revisiones.	Doctor	It is important to lead a healthy lifestyle, which includes a balanced diet, regular exercise, not smoking, managing stress, and having regular check-ups.

[Now, switch roles and practice the conversation again.]

Exercise 4

- Immobilize the injured area.

  Inmovilice el área lesionada.

  Inmovilice el área cortada.

Inmovilice el área quemada.

- Take the patient to the nearest hospital.

  Lleve al paciente al hospital más al sur.

  Lleve al paciente al hospital más lejano.

  Lleve al paciente al hospital más cercano.

- Have the emergency equipment ready.

  Tenga lejos el equipo de urgencia.

  Tenga listo el equipo de emergencia.

  Tenga fuera el equipo de primeros auxilios.

- Prepare the automated external defibrillator (AED).

  Prepare el desfibrilador externo automático (DEA).

  Prepare el desfibrilador automático externo (DAE).

  Prepare el desfibrilador externo automático (AED).

- Perform cardiopulmonary resuscitation (CPR).

  Realice la resucitación cardiopulmonar (RCP).

  Realice la reanimación cardiopulmonar (RCP).

  Realice la reanimación cardiovascular (RCV).

Exercise 5

Spanish	English
Evacue el área	Evacuate the area
Pida refuerzos si es necesario	Call for backup if necessary
Comuníquese con el centro de control de envenenamientos	Contact the poison control center
Notifique a la familia del paciente	Notify the patient's family

Learn Medical Spanish for Healthcare Professionals

BOOK

03

Cultural Competence in Healthcare and Additional Practice

Building Bridges of Understanding: Cultivating
Cultural Competence in Healthcare and Beyond!

Book 3 Description

Welcome to the third part of our series, 'Cultural Competence in Healthcare and Additional Practice.' If you have reached this point, you're on a journey to becoming an inclusive and culturally sensitive caregiver continues, enhancing your understanding and skills in medical Spanish.

This guide delves into the profound significance of cultural competence in healthcare interactions with Spanish-speaking patients. In our increasingly diverse global landscape, mastering medical Spanish goes beyond language proficiency; it fosters genuine connections and ensures equitable care.

Chapter by chapter, you'll refine your communication abilities during critical moments, such as medical emergencies, learning essential vocabulary and compassionate phrases to navigate these situations seamlessly. Real-life conversations between healthcare professionals and patients will further solidify your expertise and readiness.

Beyond language, explore the depths of Hispanic healthcare practices, understanding traditional healing methods, cultural concepts, and the nuances of the Latino family. Gain a deep appreciation for cultural diversity and the importance of building trust with patients from diverse backgrounds.

Practice exercises throughout the book will improve your pronunciation, expand your medical vocabulary by specialty, and immerse you in scenarios that enhance cultural competence. From mastering the Spanish naming system to utilizing region-specific expressions, these exercises will elevate your language abilities and cultural awareness.

In the appendices, find valuable resources including medical abbreviations, a glossary of medical Spanish terms, conjugations, and pronunciation guides, as well as a Spanish-English and English-Spanish medical dictionary for quick reference.

As you conclude this enriching journey, celebrate your milestones and accomplishments in mastering medical Spanish and cultural competence. Embrace diversity and elevate your practice as a culturally competent healthcare professional, empowering yourself to provide truly inclusive care and create meaningful connections with your Spanish-speaking patients.

Are you ready to embark on this transformative path? Let 'Cultural Competence in Healthcare and Additional Practice' be your guide to becoming a true healthcare ally, transcending language barriers and embracing diversity in medicine.

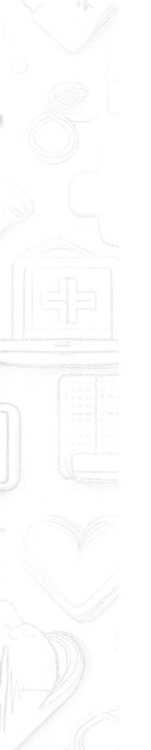

Chapter 1:
Introduction

Vivir es extraerse del corazón cada mañana una brasa de sueño para seguir creando.

Josefina Plá

This chapter will focus on vocabulary and phrases for emergency situations. In this third book, we explore the significance of cultural competence in effectively engaging with diverse people and communities. Embracing understanding and empathy, we aim to bridge differences and foster inclusivity in our global community.

Step into the realm of 'Cultural Knowledge,' immersing yourself in the rich tapestry of distinct characteristics, histories, values, and behaviors of various ethnic and cultural groups. This foundational exploration sets the stage for the thrilling next phase—'Cultural Awareness.' Here, embark on a fearless journey of self-exploration, reevaluating and reshaping pre-existing cultural attitudes.

The metamorphosis that unfolds is the very essence of fostering profound understanding and respect between cultures, extending beyond the pages of this book into life itself.

Building on this groundwork, we progress to "Cultural Sensitivity." This stage illuminates the rich diversity between cultures without imposing value judgments, emphasizing the importance of maintaining respect amidst diversity. It acknowledges and mitigates potential conflicts arising from differing customs and beliefs, crucial in our multicultural world where internal conflicts can stem from these complex intercultural interactions.

Moving forward to Cultural Competence, this stage encompasses the appreciation of diversity and respecting differences within and across cultures. It dispels the common misconception that members of the same racial, linguistic, or religious groups share a homogeneous culture. Individuals within a group, while sharing certain commonalities, embody unique cultural experiences, particularly apparent when societies merge and individuals assimilate into new environments, fostering a vibrant mix of subcultures.

Let's illustrate this with the example of healthcare. A medical professional treating a Hispanic patient must comprehend that the Hispanic culture, while united by shared historical and geographical experiences, is far from homogeneous. Each patient brings a unique set of beliefs and norms shaped by their individual experiences. Recognizing and respecting these nuances can enhance communication, promote mutual respect, and foster improved healthcare outcomes.

Dr. Maria tailored her approach to Mr. Garcia —an older patient of Mexican descent— for Type 2 Diabetes. Instead of imposing a standard diet, she consulted with a nutritionist familiar with Mexican cuisine to create a customized diet that accommodated his cultural food preferences. She also integrated his traditional belief that diseases were a divine test into her counseling, strengthening his acceptance of the diagnosis. Involving his family in the treatment process, leveraged his strong sense of familial responsibility.

Dr. Maria's ability to understand the unique aspects of Mr. Garcia's cultural background fostered improved communication, mutual respect, and effective healthcare outcomes. This example underscores the importance of recognizing that Hispanic culture, while sharing common roots, encompasses diverse individual experiences that healthcare providers must consider.

At its essence, culture is dynamic, shaped by communities or societies, influencing our worldview, norms, values, and beliefs regarding relationships, lifestyle, and environmental organization. Therefore, individuals often belong to multiple cultural groups within any nation, race, or community, each with its distinct set of norms.

"Cultural Identity" encapsulates this fluidity, illustrating an individual's connection to various groups. It's a dynamic entity that continually evolves over an individual's lifetime, reflecting diverse perspectives even among individuals identifying with the same culture. This underscores the necessity for an individualized approach in developing cultural competence.

Through this book, we aim to guide you in comprehending these intricacies and enriching your cultural competence, and promoting improved communication and understanding in healthcare and beyond.

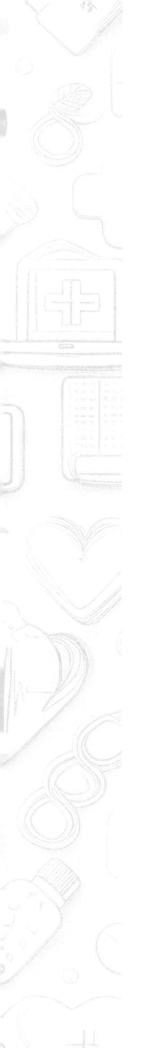

Chapter 2:
Enhancing Cultural Competence in Healthcare

Consultando entre sí y meditando, se pusieron de acuerdo, juntaron sus palabras y su pensamiento.

Popol Wuj

In today's diverse healthcare landscape, healthcare professionals must provide culturally competent care. This chapter focuses on refining cultural competence in healthcare, specifically for Spanish-speaking patients. It covers topics such as cultural diversity, effective communication strategies, understanding common patient responses, and the Spanish naming system. By the end of this chapter, readers will have a deeper understanding of how to provide culturally competent care to Spanish-speaking patients.

Cultural diversity in healthcare

The Hispanic population comprises individuals with diverse cultural origins and life experiences. While the term "Hispanic" may be used to refer to people with roots in Latin America or Spain, this group embraces a wide range of cultures, languages, and traditions. Healthcare professionals must understand that the Hispanic population is diverse, with cultural differences can significantly impact healthcare outcomes.

In certain Hispanic cultures, family members often play a pivotal role in healthcare decision-making. It is common to seek their input before patients decide on treatment options or involve them directly in care provision. Diverse cultural groups may strongly prefer traditional therapies or hold specific beliefs about illness causes and treatments. For instance, some Hispanic patients might prefer herbal remedies or be cautious with medications, often turning to natural treatments before seeking medical help. Additionally, religious beliefs often shape how Hispanics approach healthcare, underscoring the need for providers to respect and understand these beliefs.

For example, in Mexican culture, curanderos (traditional healers) use herbal remedies, spiritual rituals, and massages for healing, often consulted before medical professionals, particularly in rural areas. Similarly, in Puerto Rico, espiritismo (spiritism) involves seeking guidance and spiritual cleansing from mediums or healers.

Now, let's discuss an important term: Interculturality in Health. This concept denotes recognizing, respecting, and understanding the socio-cultural diversity among communities and their healthcare practices to enhance public health. Effective dialogue and communication among doctors, patients, family members, healthcare personnel with different cultural backgrounds are essential for addressing local development issues and healthcare needs. This approach not only combats discrimination but also promotes the right to health for marginalized groups, leading to more effective health interventions.

Latin America hosts approximately 42 million indigenous people across numerous distinct ethnic groups. The countries like Mexico, Guatemala, Peru, and Bolivia have the largest indigenous populations, totaling around 34 million. These indigenous groups preserve their languages, traditions, and worldviews alongside Spanish, influencing their healthcare practices. Understanding and respecting the traditional practices and knowledge of these communities is essential for improving the health and overall well-being of Indigenous populations in the region.

Some of the most prominent indigenous groups include:

- Mexico: Home to 68 recognized indigenous groups, including the Nahuas, Mayas, Mixtecos, and Zapotecos.
- Guatemala: Predominantly inhabited by the Maya, Garífuna, Xinka, and Mestizo peoples.
- Peru: Quechua and Aymara are the primary indigenous groups, with significant communities in the Andean region.
- Bolivia: Dominated by the Quechua and Aymara peoples, who represent a large part of the country's indigenous population.
- Brazil: Boasts over 300 indigenous groups, including the Guaraní, Yanomami, and Tikuna.
- Colombia: Hosts more than 100 indigenous groups, including the Wayuu, Nasa, and Embera.

These examples underscore the cultural diversity within the Hispanic population and highlight the importance of cultural competence:

Mexican Americans	Puerto Ricans	Cuban Americans
Largest Hispanic subgroup in the United States.	Their culture is a blend of Taíno, African, and Spanish influences, leading to specific beliefs about health and wellness.	They are a smaller Hispanic subgroup in the United States, and their culture is heavily influenced by Spanish and Afro-Caribbean traditions.
Their culture is heavily influenced by indigenous and Spanish traditions, and they may have specific beliefs about health and illness.	They may use "susto", a condition caused by a frightening experience, to explain certain illnesses.	They may hold specific beliefs about health, Curanderismo and wellness, such as the use of santería, a syncretic religion that blends African and Catholic beliefs.
They often emphasize the importance of "hot" and "cold" foods and how they can impact health.		

To illustrate the cultural diversity within the Hispanic population, consider the following case study:

Case study:

- **Scenario**: Mrs. Lopez, a 45-year-old woman from Guatemala, visits the clinic with her teenage daughter. Mrs. Lopez prefers to use traditional herbal remedies for minor illnesses and relies on her religious beliefs for health guidance. Her daughter, on the other hand, has embraced modern healthcare practices.

- **Approach**: The healthcare provider, understanding their cultural background, engages in a respectful conversation about their health beliefs. The provider suggests integrating some herbal remedies with prescribed medications for Mrs. Lopez, explaining their potential interactions. For the daughter, the provider offers a more conventional treatment plan, ensuring she feels comfortable and respected.

- **Outcome**: By acknowledging and respecting their cultural beliefs, the provider builds trust with both patients. Mrs. Lopez is more willing to adhere to the prescribed treatment, knowing her cultural practices are respected, and her daughter feels understood and supported in her healthcare choices.

Understanding the cultural diversity among Hispanics is essential for providing culturally competent care in healthcare settings. By recognizing and respecting cultural differences, healthcare professionals can better engage with patients, build trust, and ultimately improve health outcomes.

Providing culturally competent care for Spanish-speaking patients

Providing culturally competent care for Spanish-speaking patients requires healthcare professionals to understand and respect their patients' cultural backgrounds. Cultural competence involves being aware of cultural differences and how they can impact healthcare, as well as tailoring care to meet the unique needs of each patient.

One way that medical doctors can improve their understanding of Hispanic culture is by working with bilingual staff or medical interpreters. These professionals can help bridge the language barrier and ensure that patients receive accurate information and understand their treatment options. In addition, medical professionals can take the time to learn key phrases in Spanish, such as greetings, medical terms, and common phrases used during medical consultations.

Here are some more examples of different Hispanic cultures and their beliefs in medical care:

Ecuadorian Americans	Dominican Americans	Colombian Americans
They may believe in "mal aire," which is a condition caused by exposure to cold or wind.	They may have a belief in "mal de ojo," which is a condition caused by being looked at by someone with envy or jealousy.	They may beliebe in "limpias," which is a form of spiritual cleansing that is used to rid the body of negative energy.
They may also use natural remedies, such as herbs or plant extracts, for common illnesses or seek treatment from traditional healers.	They may also have a strong belief in the healing power of prayer or use natural remedies, such as herbs and teas.	"Susto" is a condition caused by trauma that can cause both physical and mental health problems.

Real-life scenario:

- **Scenario**: Dr. Rodriguez, an oncologist, is treating Lucia —a 50-year-old woman from El Salvador— who has been diagnosed with breast cancer. Lucia speaks limited English and is deeply rooted in her Salvadoran cultural practices. During the initial consultation, Lucia shares her belief in using natural remedies and prayers for healing, expressing hesitation about chemotherapy.

- **Approach**: Dr. Rodriguez respects Lucia's beliefs and explains the diagnosis and treatment options in simple Spanish. He acknowledges her preference for natural remedies and suggests incorporating them alongside conventional treatments to ensure comprehensive care. Dr. Rodriguez emphasizes that the combination of natural and medical treatments can improve her chances of recovery.

  - ⊛ Dr. Rodriguez collaborates with a local herbalist from Lucia's community. Together, they discuss safe natural remedies Lucia to complement chemotherapy. This approach ensures that Lucia feels her cultural beliefs are respected while receiving holistic care.

⊙ Additionally, Dr. Rodriguez arranges for a support group of Spanish-speaking cancer survivors to meet with Lucia. These survivors share their experiences and strategies for balancing traditional practices with medical treatments, offering peer support that reduces Lucia's isolation and strengthens her resolve to undergo chemotherapy.

- **Outcome**: By integrating Lucia's cultural beliefs with her medical treatment plan, Dr. Rodriguez builds a strong rapport and trust. Lucia feels respected and supported, leading to her increased adherence to the treatment plan. This collaborative approach effectively manages her breast cancer, combining the benefits of both natural remedies and chemotherapy.

This scenario highlights the importance of cultural competence in healthcare. Dr. Rodriguez's recognition and respect for Lucia's cultural background enabled him to provide personalized care that met her unique needs, resulting in improved health outcomes.

Effective communication strategies for Spanish-speaking patients

Navigating effective communication with Spanish-speaking patients fosters understanding and enhance patient care outcomes. Various strategies can be used to overcome language and cultural barriers, promoting clearer interactions and establishing trust between healthcare providers and their patients.

- Use simple and clear language.
- Speak slowly and enunciating clearly.
- Avoid medical jargon and technical terms.
- Utilize visual aids such as diagrams or illustrations.
- Check for understanding by asking patients to repeat or summarize information.
- Employ interpreters or bilingual staff when necessary.
- Use culturally appropriate nonverbal communication, such as eye contact and hand gestures.
- Be mindful of language barriers and adapt communication strategies accordingly.
- Discuss sexuality openly and informatively, particularly with adolescents, while considering cultural taboos.
- Focus on education about STDs and contraception.
- Highlight the higher rates of new HIV infections among Latino males and females compared to white counterparts.
- Emphasize the importance of awareness and prevention strategies.
- Explain the optional yet crucial nature of rectal exams to Hispanic men, addressing cultural concerns about the procedure.

- Highlight the significance of early cancer detection, given higher rates of advanced-stage diagnoses and related complications among Latinos.

Understanding common patient responses

Healthcare providers must understand how patients might respond in various scenarios and be prepared to react appropriately, as this improves the quality of care and patient satisfaction. Some common patient responses in Spanish include:

"Sí" (Yes)

"No" (No)

"No lo sé" (I don't know)

"Me duele aquí" (It hurts here)

"Estoy mareado/ atontado/ aturdido" (I am dizzy)

"Tengo calor" (I am hot)

"Tengo frío" (I am cold)

"Tengo hambre" (I am hungry)

"Tengo sed" (I am thirsty)

"No puedo respirar" (I can't breathe)

"Me siento débil" (I feel weak)

"Me siento enfermo" (I feel sick)

"Me siento cansado" (I feel tired)

"Me siento mejor" (I feel better)

"Me siento peor" (I feel worse)

"Me duele la cabeza" (I have a headache)

"Me siento triste" (I feel sad)

"Me siento ansioso/a" (I feel anxious)

"Me falta el aire" (I am short of breath)

"Me duele el estómago/ Me duele la panza/ Me duele la barriga" (I have stomach pain)

"Me duele el pecho" (I have chest pain)

"Me duele la espalda" (I have back pain)

"Me duele la garganta" (I have a sore throat)

"Me duele la pierna" (I have leg pain)

"Me duele el brazo" (I have arm pain)

"Me duele el oído" (I have ear pain)

"Me duele el diente" (I have a toothache)

"Me duele el cuerpo" (I have body pain)

"Tengo un resfriado" (I have a cold)

"Tengo la gripe" (I have the flu)

"Tengo alergia a" (I have allergy to)

"Tengo una infección" (I have an infection)

"Tengo una herida aquí" (I have a wound here)

"Me fracture/ partí/ quebré/ rompí el brazo" (I broke my arm)

"Gracias" (Thank you)

"De nada" (You're welcome)

"Lo siento" (I'm sorry)

"No hay problema" (No problem)

"Adiós" (Goodbye)

Understanding the Spanish naming system and identifying common errors

Healthcare professionals benefit from understanding the nuances of the Spanish naming system when interacting with Spanish-speaking patients. Across different Hispanic cultures, variations in surname conventions are notable. For example, in Mexican and Colombian cultures, it is common for individuals to use both their paternal and maternal surnames, whereas Cuban and Puerto Rican cultures often use only the paternal surname.

Moreover, Spanish-speaking patients may sometimes make errors when providing their names, such as omitting a surname, using a non-legally recognized surname, or providing an incorrect spelling. Healthcare professionals should take the time to confirm and verify the patient's name, using identification documents, to ensure accurate medical record keeping.

Healthcare providers should also consider cultural differences that can influence naming practices. For example, some Hispanic cultures may have different naming traditions for children, such as using family names or names of religious significance. Healthcare professionals should be sensitive to these cultural nuances, respecting patients' preferences when documenting their names in medical records.

Below are examples illustrating differences in the Spanish naming system among different Hispanic cultures:

Region	Naming system
Mexican Americans	Often use both paternal and maternal surnames, such as Rodriguez Garcia.
Puerto Ricans	Typically use only the paternal surname, such as Rodriguez.
Cuban Americans	May use both paternal and maternal surnames, but the paternal surname is typically listed first, such as Rodriguez Garcia
Salvadoran Americans	Often use both paternal and maternal surnames, but the maternal surname is typically listed first, such as Garcia Rodriguez
Dominican Americans	Typically use both paternal and maternal surnames, such as Rodriguez Garcia, but may also use a maternal surname as a middle name, such as Rodriguez de Garcia
Colombian Americans	Often use both paternal and maternal surnames, such as Garcia Rodriguez
Ecuadorian Americans	May use both paternal and maternal surnames, but the paternal surname is typically listed first, such as Rodriguez Garcia
Venezuelan Americans	May use both paternal and maternal surnames, but the paternal surname is typically listed first, such as Rodriguez Garcia
Peruvian Americans	May use both paternal and maternal surnames, such as Garcia Rodriguez
Argentinian Americans	May use both paternal and maternal surnames, but may reverse the order of the surnames, listing the maternal surname first, such as Garcia Rodriguez

Healthcare professionals must grasp the intricacies of the Spanish naming system when interacting with Spanish-speaking patients. By acknowledging cultural variations, providers can strengthen relationships and deliver culturally sensitive care effectively.

Key takeaways

- Recognizing cultural diversity among Hispanics is essential for providing culturally competent care.
- Communicating in Spanish and understanding cultural differences can improve healthcare outcomes.

- Using simple language, visual aids, and nonverbal communication improves communication strategies.

- Healthcare professionals should be aware of common patient responses in Spanish and how to respond appropriately.

- Understanding the Spanish naming system and common errors made by Spanish-speaking patients can improve the accuracy of patient information.

Exercises

Exercise 1

Choose the correct answer for the following questions:

1. What is an effective communication strategy for Spanish-speaking patients?

   A) Using complex medical terminology

   B) Speaking quickly

   C) Using visual aids such as diagrams or illustrations

   D) Not checking for understanding

2. Why is it important for healthcare professionals to understand the cultural diversity among Hispanics?

   A) It is not important

   B) To provide effective care that is tailored to the unique needs of each patient

   C) To discriminate against certain cultures

   D) To provide ineffective care

3. What is one way that medical doctors can improve their understanding of Hispanic culture?

   A) Avoiding working with bilingual staff

   B) Speaking English only

   C) Learning key phrases in Spanish

   D) Disrespecting patients' cultural beliefs

4. What is the typical naming convention for Cuban Americans?

   A) Typically use both paternal and maternal surnames, with the paternal surname listed first.

   B) Typically use only the paternal surname.

   C) Typically use both paternal and maternal surnames, but the maternal surname is typically listed first.

   D) Typically use both paternal and maternal surnames, with the maternal surname listed first.

5. Why is it important for healthcare professionals to understand common patient responses in Spanish?

    A) It is not important

    B) To provide inaccurate information

    C) To ignore the patient's concerns

    D) To respond appropriately to certain questions or situations

Exercise 2

Fill in the blanks with the appropriate word(s) from the chapter:

1. Understanding cultural diversity among Hispanics can help healthcare professionals provide more _____ care that is tailored to the unique needs of each patient.

2. One way that medical doctors can improve their understanding of Hispanic culture is by working with _____ or medical interpreters.

3. _____ are often consulted before a patient makes a decision about treatment or may play an active role in the care process in some Hispanic cultures.

4. Healthcare professionals working with Spanish-speaking patients must understand the Spanish naming system to ensure accurate _____.

5. Effective communication is essential in healthcare, especially when working with _____ patients.

Words: Spanish speaking, bilingual staff, medical record keeping, Family members, Effective

Exercise 3

Indicate whether the following statements are true or false:

1. Healthcare professionals should use complex medical terminology when communicating with Spanish-speaking patients.

2. Understanding the cultural diversity among Hispanics is not important when providing healthcare.

3. Using visual aids such as diagrams or illustrations is an effective communication strategy for Spanish-speaking patients.

4. Healthcare professionals should disregard the cultural beliefs and values of their patients.

5. The typical naming convention for Mexican Americans is to use only the paternal surname.

Exercise 4

Match the Hispanic culture with their typical naming convention (*these are not in order*):

Hispanic Culture	Naming convention
Mexican Americans	Typically use only the paternal surname.
Puerto Ricans	Typically use both paternal and maternal surnames, with the paternal surname listed first.
Cuban Americans	Typically use both paternal and maternal surnames, but the maternal surname is typically listed first.
Salvadoran Americans	Typically use both paternal and maternal surnames, with the paternal surname listed first.

Exercise 5

Provide a short answer for the following questions:

1. Why is it important for healthcare professionals to check for understanding when communicating with Spanish-speaking patients?

2. What is an example of a cultural difference that may impact healthcare outcomes for Hispanic patients?

3. What are some effective communication strategies for Spanish-speaking patients?

4. Why is it important for healthcare professionals to understand common patient responses in Spanish?

5. What is the typical naming convention for Colombian Americans?

Answer key

Exercise 1

1. What is an effective communication strategy for Spanish-speaking patients?

    A) Using complex medical terminology

    B) Speaking quickly

    C) Using visual aids such as diagrams or illustrations

    D) Not checking for understanding

2. Why is it important for healthcare professionals to understand the cultural diversity among Hispanics?

    A) It is not important

    B) To provide effective care that is tailored to the unique needs of each patient

    C) To discriminate against certain cultures

    D) To provide ineffective care

3. What is one way that medical doctors can improve their understanding of Hispanic culture?

    A) Avoiding working with bilingual staff

    B) Speaking English only

    C) Learning key phrases in Spanish

    D) Disrespecting patients' cultural beliefs

4. What is the typical naming convention for Cuban Americans?

    A) Typically use both paternal and maternal surnames, with the paternal surname listed first.

    B) Typically use only the paternal surname.

    C) Typically use both paternal and maternal surnames, but the maternal surname is typically listed first.

    D) Typically use both paternal and maternal surnames, with the maternal surname listed first.

5. Why is it important for healthcare professionals to understand common patient responses in Spanish?

    A) It is not important

    B) To provide inaccurate information

    C) To ignore the patient's concerns

    D) To respond appropriately to certain questions or situations

Exercise 2

1. Understanding cultural diversity among Hispanics can help healthcare professionals provide more **effective** care that is tailored to the unique needs of each patient.

2. One way that medical doctors can improve their understanding of Hispanic culture is by working with **bilingual** staff or medical interpreters.

3. **Family members** are often consulted before a patient makes a decision about treatment or may play an active role in the care process in some Hispanic cultures.

4. Healthcare professionals working with Spanish-speaking patients must understand the Spanish naming system to ensure accurate **medical record keeping**.

5. Effective communication is essential in healthcare, especially when working with **Spanish-speaking** patients.

Exercise 3

1. False

2. False

3. True

4. False

5. False

Exercise 4

Hispanic Culture	Naming convention
Mexican Americans	Typically use both paternal and maternal surnames, with the paternal surname listed first.
Puerto Ricans	Typically use only the paternal surname
Cuban Americans	Typically use both paternal and maternal surnames, with the paternal surname listed first.
Salvadoran Americans	Typically use both paternal and maternal surnames, but the maternal surname is typically listed first.

Exercise 5

1. What is an example of a cultural difference that may impact healthcare outcomes for Hispanic patients?

Answer: One example of a cultural difference that may impact healthcare outcomes for Hispanic patients is the preference for traditional healing practices over Western medicine, which may lead to noncompliance with treatment plans.

2. What are some effective communication strategies for Spanish-speaking patients?

Answer: Effective communication strategies for Spanish-speaking patients include using simple and clear language, speaking slowly and enunciating clearly, avoiding medical jargon and technical terms, using visual aids such as diagrams or illustrations, checking for understanding by asking patients to repeat or summarize information, and using interpreters or bilingual staff when necessary.

3. Why is it important for healthcare professionals to understand common patient responses in Spanish?

Answer: It is important for healthcare professionals to understand common patient responses in Spanish to respond appropriately to certain questions or situations, which can help ensure accurate diagnosis and treatment.

4. What is the typical naming convention for Colombian Americans?

Answer: The typical naming convention for Colombian Americans is to use both paternal and maternal surnames, such as Garcia Rodriguez.

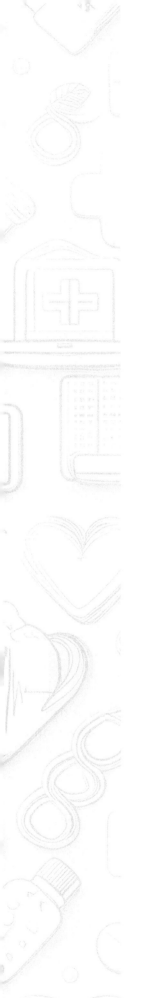

Chapter 3:
Cultural Concepts in Hispanic Healthcare

La atención médica efectiva requiere una comprensión de los conceptos y prácticas culturales.

Elena Rios

In this chapter, we explore relevant cultural concepts for healthcare professionals working with Hispanic patients. Topics include building trust in the Hispanic community, traditional healing practices such as Curanderismo and Chamanismo, common ailments like empacho, mal de ojo, and susto, navigating formal and familiar healthcare settings in, cultural considerations in the U.S. healthcare system, the importance of the Latino family in healthcare, and finally, key takeaways and exercises to reinforce your understanding of these concepts.

Building trust

Building trust is foundational within the Hispanic community. Hispanics value interpersonal relationships greatly, and building a relationship with your patient can go a long way towards developing trust. To achieve this, it is important to take the time to actively listen to patients, address their concerns thoroughly and explain procedures and treatments clearly. Being open to questions and demonstrating respect and cultural sensitivity are also integral when caring for Hispanic patients.

Traditional healing practices: Curanderismo and Chamanismo

Curanderismo and Chamanismo are traditional healing practices that are still used by many Hispanics today. While both involve the use of herbs and natural remedies, they have distinct differences. Curanderismo is a Mexican folk healing practice that combines indigenous healing methods with Catholicism, addressing physical, emotional, and spiritual ailments. On the other hand, Chamanismo originated in the Andes and Amazon regions of South America as a spiritual practice using shamanic rituals and ceremonies to heal both physical and emotional ailments.

While these practices share similarities, they also present notable differences:

Similarities	Differences
Rooted in indigenous traditions and beliefs.	Curanderismo primarily focuses on healing physical, emotional, and spiritual ailments, while Chamanismo is primarily focused on spiritual healing.
Based on the idea of maintaining balance and harmony between the body, mind, and spirit.	Curanderismo is heavily influenced by Catholicism, while Chamanismo has its roots in indigenous beliefs from the Andes and Amazon regions of South America.
View illness as a result of imbalance, either physical or spiritual.	Curanderismo practitioners are known as curanderos, while Chamanismo practitioners are known as shamans.
Use natural remedies such as herbs and plants to promote healing.	Curanderismo often involves the use of objects such as candles, amulets, and crosses in rituals, while Chamanismo incorporates music and dance.
Emphasize the importance of spiritual connection and involve rituals and ceremonies to achieve this connection.	Curanderismo is more prevalent in Mexico and other parts of Central America, while Chamanismo is more prevalent in South America.

While both Curanderismo and Chamanismo share some commonalities, such as a focus on natural remedies, spiritual connection, and the importance of maintaining balance, they also have some distinct differences, such as their primary focus, cultural roots, and specific practices.

Understanding common ailments: empacho, mal de ojo, susto and culebrilla

Several common ailments in Hispanic communities have spiritual and cultural roots that healthcare professionals must understand to provide effective care to Hispanic patients. Some of the most common ailments include empacho, mal de ojo, susto, and culebrilla.

Empacho	Empacho is a condition caused by overeating or eating something that is difficult to digest; it can cause stomach pain, nausea, and vomiting. The traditional treatment for empacho involves a curandero, or traditional healer, who will use massage techniques to help move the food through the digestive system. For example, a curandero may use a technique called "sobar el estómago", which involves massaging the stomach in circular movements to help ease the symptoms. In Cuba and other regions, the curandero can massage the legs "sobar las piernas", massage the back "la espalda" or massage the arms "los brazos".
Mal de ojo	Mal de ojo, or the evil eye, is a condition believed to be caused by a person with negative energy or bad intentions. It can cause headaches, stomach pain, and general malaise. The traditional treatment for mal de ojo involves a curandero who will use various methods to remove the bad energy from the patient. For example, a curandero may use an egg to remove the negative energy or perform a cleansing ritual involving herbs and prayer.
Susto	Susto attributed to trauma or fright, leading to diverse physical and emotional symptoms like insomnia, loss of appetite, and anxiety. Traditional treatment involves a curandero employing methods such as cleansing rituals or herbal remedies to restore the patient's well-being by reclaiming their lost soul.
Culebrilla	Culebrilla —also known as herpes zoster or shingles— is a viral infection that results in a painful rash. It is caused by the varicella-zoster virus, the same virus that causes chickenpox. After a person recovers from chickenpox, the virus remains dormant in the body and can reactivate years later as shingles.

Healthcare professionals should be aware of these common ailments and approach them with cultural sensitivity and respect. While these ailments may have spiritual and cultural roots, it is also important to address any physical symptoms that may be present and provide appropriate medical treatment as necessary.

Navigating Formal and Familiar Settings in Hispanic Healthcare

Hispanics in the USA: cultural considerations in healthcare

When interacting with Hispanic patients in the United States, healthcare professionals must navigate diverse cultural backgrounds to ensure effective care. In the U.S., all Hispanics come from a variety of countries and traditions, and it is important to understand the specific cultural norms and values of the patient you are working with. For instance, family plays a significant role in Hispanic culture, so involving family members in healthcare decisions can enhance patient engagement and satisfaction.

Also, it is important to recognize the unique cultural norms of specific Hispanic groups, such as Mexican Americans, Puerto Ricans, or Cuban-Americans, to deliver culturally sensitive healthcare services effectively.

Moreover, Hispanic patients often have common complaints about the U.S. healthcare system, and providers should be aware of these during their interactions:

- Doctors prioritize typing on the computer or sending patients for MRI scans instead of conducting physical exams.
- Doctors frequently avoid making eye contact and fail to remember patients' names.
- There is a perception that patients without payment are left to die.
- Patients feel they are treated as diseases rather than as human beings.
- Much of the work is done by nurses or assistants rather than the doctor.
- Consultations often last only one minute.
- Accessing the doctor's contact number is often impossible.
- Dealing with health insurance companies is challenging, and nearly 1 in 5 Hispanic Americans lack health insurance, a rate almost three times higher than that of Anglos.

Addressing these concerns can help improve the patient-provider relationship and ensure better healthcare outcomes for Hispanic patients.

Defining Hispanic or Latino: understanding identity

The terms Hispanic and Latino are often used interchangeably, but they carry distinct meanings that are important for healthcare professionals working with these communities.

Hispanic refers to individuals who come from Spanish-speaking countries, including Spain and many countries in Latin America, South and Central America, as well as the Caribbean. On the other hand, Latino includes people who come from Latin America, encompassing Spanish-speaking countries Brazil, where the official language is Portuguese.

Not all Hispanics or Latinos share the same cultural background or identity. Many also identify with their specific country of origin and may have strong ties to that culture. For instance, someone from Puerto Rico may identify as Hispanic or Latino, but they may also identify specifically as Puerto Rican and have a strong connection to Puerto Rican culture and traditions.

Identity is complex across all cultures, and it is important to be aware of their patients' diverse identities and backgrounds. By learning about their patients' cultural norms and values, healthcare providers can offer more effective and culturally sensitive care.

Additionally, recognize that identity is fluid with individuals embracing different aspects at various stages of life. For example, a person who was born in Mexico and raised in the United States may identify as Mexican American or Hispanic, while also feeling a strong connection to American culture. All identities are valid and should be respected.

By embracing and respecting the diverse identities and cultural backgrounds of Hispanic and Latino patients, healthcare professionals can foster trust, enhance communication, and ultimately improve health outcomes.

The importance of the Latino family in healthcare

The Latino family plays a significant role in healthcare decisions. It is common for family members to be involved in healthcare decisions, and they may also be responsible for providing care for their loved ones at home. Healthcare professionals should actively engage family members in the care process while remaining mindful of the unique family dynamics and cultural norms involved.

Key takeaways

- Build trust in the Hispanic community by taking the time to listen to your patient, being open to answering questions, and being respectful and culturally sensitive.

- Emphasize spirituality and the connection between the body, mind, and spirit in traditional healing practices like Curanderismo and Chamanismo.

- Recognize that empacho, mal de ojo, and susto are common ailments in Hispanic communities that have spiritual and cultural roots.

- Divide Hispanic healthcare settings into formal and familiar settings, maintaining professionalism and respect in formal settings while using informal language in familiar ones.

- Be aware of the variety of countries and cultural backgrounds among Hispanics in the United States, and involve family members in healthcare decisions whenever possible.

Exercises

Exercise 1: Building trust

Match the following actions with the strategies to build trust with Hispanic patients:

Actions	Strategies
1. Take the time to listen to your patient	a. Develop a personal relationship with your patient
2. Address their concerns	b. Use informal language in familiar settings
3. Explain procedures and treatments in an easy-to-understand way	c. Involve family members in healthcare decisions
4. Be respectful and culturally sensitive	d. Be open to answering any questions your patient may have

Exercise 2: Traditional healing practices

Fill in the blanks with the appropriate words or phrases from the table:

Curanderismo is a Mexican folk healing practice that combines _____ healing methods with _____. It is often used to treat physical, emotional, and spiritual ailments. On the other hand, Chamanismo is a spiritual practice that originated in the _____ regions of South America. It involves the use of shamanic rituals and ceremonies to heal both physical and emotional ailments. While both practices have their roots in indigenous traditions and beliefs, Curanderismo is primarily focused on healing physical, emotional, and spiritual ailments, while Chamanismo focuses mainly on _____ healing.

Exercise 3: Common ailments

Choose the appropriate treatment for each of the following common ailments:

1. Empacho

    a. A curandero will use massage techniques to help move the food through the digestive system.

    b. A curandero will use an egg to draw out the negative energy.

    c. A curandero will use various methods to help the patient recover their lost soul.

2. Mal de ojo

    a. A curandero will use massage techniques to help move the food through the digestive system.

    b. A curandero will use an egg to draw out the negative energy.

    c. A curandero will use various methods to remove the bad energy from the patient.

3. Susto

    a. A curandero will use massage techniques to help move the food through the digestive system.

    b. A curandero will use an egg to draw out the negative energy.

    c. A curandero will use various methods to help the patient recover their lost soul.

Exercise 4: Cultural differences

Match the following cultural norms or values with the Hispanic community they are commonly associated with:

Cultural Norms/Values Hispanic Community

    1. Strong emphasis on family and community

    2. Influence of Catholicism in healing practices

    3. More prevalent in Mexico and Central America

    4. More prevalent in South America

    5. Different cultural norms and values based on specific country of origin

    a. Mexican Americans

    b. Puerto Ricans

    c. Curanderismo

    d. Chamanismo

    e. Hispanics/Latinos in general

Exercise 5: Cultural sensitivity

Match the following actions with the strategies for demonstrating cultural sensitivity in healthcare:

Actions	Strategies
1. Be aware of cultural differences	a. Use formal language in formal settings
2. Involve family members in healthcare decisions	b. Understand the specific cultural norms and values of the patient
3. Use appropriate language and terminology	c. Be aware of the cultural significance of certain practices or objects
4. Respect personal space and touch boundaries	d. Recognize that the patient's cultural background may influence their health beliefs and practices

Answer key

Exercise 1: Building trust

1. Develop a personal relationship with your patient (a)

2. Be open to answering any questions your patient may have (d)

3. Explain procedures and treatments in an easy-to-understand way (b)

4. Be respectful and culturally sensitive (c)

Exercise 2: Traditional Healing Practices

Curanderismo is a Mexican folk healing practice that combines **Mexican folk** healing methods with **Catholicism**. It is often used to treat physical, emotional, and spiritual ailments. On the other hand, Chamanismo is a spiritual practice that originated in the **Andes and Amazon** regions of South America. It involves the use of shamanic rituals and ceremonies to heal both physical and emotional ailments. While both practices have their roots in indigenous traditions and beliefs, Curanderismo is primarily focused on healing physical, emotional, and spiritual ailments, while Chamanismo focuses mainly on spiritual healing.

Exercise 3: Common ailments

1. Empacho - a. A curandero will use massage techniques to help move the food through the digestive system.

2. Mal de ojo - c. A curandero will use various methods to remove the bad energy from the patient.

3. Susto - c. A curandero will use various methods to help the patient recover their lost soul.

Exercise 4: Cultural differences

1. Strong emphasis on family and community - e. Hispanics/Latinos in general

2. Influence of Catholicism in healing practices - c. Curanderismo

3. More prevalent in Mexico and Central America - a. Mexican Americans

4. More prevalent in South America - d. Chamanismo

5. Different cultural norms and values based on specific country of origin - b. Puerto Ricans

Exercise 5: Cultural sensitivity

Actions	Strategies
1. Be aware of cultural differences	b. Understand the specific cultural norms and values of the patient

Actions	Strategies
2. Involve family members in healthcare decisions	d. Recognize that the patient's cultural background may influence their health beliefs and practices
3. Use appropriate language and terminology	a. Use formal language in formal settings
4. Respect personal space and touch boundaries	c. Be aware of the cultural significance of certain practices or objects

Chapter 4:
Additional Practice Exercises

Solo los que tienen la paciencia de hacer cosas simples con precisión y dedicación alcanzarán la habilidad de hacer cosas difíciles con facilidad y excelencia.

James J. Corbett

Congratulations on making it this far in your journey to learn medical Spanish! In this chapter, we will explore additional practice exercises that will help you reinforce what you have learned so far and improve your skills in speaking and understanding medical Spanish. These exercises will challenge you to apply your knowledge in diverse contexts, improve your listening comprehension, and expand your vocabulary in an enjoyable and engaging manner. Let's dive in!

Spanish pronunciation exercises

To effectively speak Spanish, you must have a good grasp of its pronunciation. It not only ensures that you are understood but also helps you sound more natural and confident. This section provides a few exercises that can aid you in perfecting your Spanish pronunciation.

Exercise 1: Vowels

As we mentioned in previous chapters, Spanish vowels differ from English vowels in that they have a consistent sound. The five vowels in Spanish are: a, e, i, o, and u. To help you master these sounds, try the following exercises:

- First, begin by saying each vowel sound slowly and clearly: a, e, i, o, u.

- Next, try pronouncing these vowel sounds in various combinations, such as ae, ei, io, ou, and au.

- Finally, practice saying words that contain each vowel sound, like casa (house), perro (dog), libro (book), ojo (eye), and uva (grape).

Exercise 2: Consonants

Although many Spanish consonants sound the same as their English counterparts, some have distinct pronunciations. Here are a few exercises to assist you in correctly pronouncing Spanish consonants:

- To practice the "rr" sound, try saying "perro" (dog) and "ferrocarril" (railroad) slowly while rolling your tongue.

- To practice the "j" sound, emphasize the "j" sound while saying "joven" (young) and "jardín" (garden) slowly.

- To practice the "ñ" sound, emphasize the "ñ" sound while saying "mañana" (tomorrow) and "muñeca" (doll) slowly.

Medical Spanish vocabulary and exercises by specialty

Depending on your specialty, you may need to be familiar with specific medical terms that extends beyond basics. Here are some useful examples:

Cardiología / Cardiology

1. Infarto de miocardio (myocardial infarction): in-FAR-toh deh myoh-KAR-dyoh

2. Arritmia ventricular (ventricular arrhythmia): ah-REE-mee-ah ven-tree-KOO-lar

3. Cateterismo cardíaco (cardiac catheterization): kah-teh-teh-REES-moh kar-DEE-ah-koh

4. Insuficiencia cardíaca congestiva (congestive heart failure): een-soo-fee-SYEN-syah kar-DEE-ah-kah kon-HES-tee-vah

5. Angioplastia coronaria (coronary angioplasty): ahn-hee-oh-PLAS-tee-ah koh-roh-NAH-ree-ah

6. Fibrilación ventricular (ventricular fibrillation): fee-bree-lah-SYON ven-tree-KOO-lar

7. Marcapasos bicameral (dual-chamber pacemaker): mar-kah-PAH-sohs bee-kah-MEH-rahl

8. Ecocardiografía transesofágica (transesophageal echocardiography): eh-koh-kar-dee-oh-GRAH-fee-ah trans-eh-soh-FAH-hee-kah

9. Hipertensión sistémica (systemic hypertension): ee-per-ten-SYON see-STEM-ee-kah

10. Soplo cardíaco sistólico (systolic heart murmur): SOH-ploh kar-DEE-ah-koh see-STO-lee-koh

Pediatría / Pediatrics

1. Vacuna de rotavirus (rotavirus vaccine): bah-KOO-nah deh roh-tah-VEE-roos

2. Diarrea aguda (acute diarrhea): dee-ah-RREH-ah ah-GOO-dah

3. Asma bronquial (bronchial asthma): AHS-mah bron-KEE-ahl

4. Varicela zoster (varicella-zoster): vah-ree-SEH-lah ZOS-tehr

5. Bronquiolitis obliterante (obliterative bronchiolitis): bron-kee-oh-LEE-tees oh-blee-teh-RAHN-teh

6. Sarampión (measles): sah-rahm-PYON

7. Otitis media aguda (acute otitis media): oh-TEE-tees MEH-dee-ah ah-GOO-dah

8. Escarlatina estreptocócica (streptococcal scarlet fever): es-kar-lah-TEE-nah es-trep-toh-KOH-see-kah

9. Cólico infantil (infant colic): KOH-lee-koh een-fan-TEEL

10. Tos ferina (whooping cough): tos feh-REE-nah

Ginecología y Obstetricia / Gynecology and Obstetrics

1. Embarazo ectópico (ectopic pregnancy): em-bah-RAH-soh ek-TOP-ee-koh

2. Cesárea de emergencia (emergency cesarean section): seh-SAH-reh-ah deh eh-mer-HEN-syah

3. Parto prematuro (preterm birth): PAHR-toh preh-mah-TOO-roh

4. Menstruación irregular (irregular menstruation): men-stroo-AH-syon ee-reh-goo-LAR

5. Endometriosis severa (severe endometriosis): en-doh-meh-tree-OH-sees seh-VEH-rah

6. Menopausia precoz (premature menopause): meh-noh-PAW-syah preh-KOHZ

7. Anticonceptivo hormonal (hormonal contraceptive): an-tee-kon-sehp-TEE-voh or-MOH-nahl

8. Ecografía doppler (doppler ultrasound): eh-koh-grah-FEE-ah DOP-ler

9. Preeclampsia severa (severe preeclampsia): preh-eh-KLAMP-see-ah seh-VEH-rah

10. Aborto espontáneo recurrente (recurrent miscarriage): ah-BOR-toh es-pon-TAH-neh-oh reh-KOOR-ehn-the

Neurología / Neurology

1. Migraña crónica (chronic migraine): mee-GRAH-nyah KROH-nee-kah

2. Accidente cerebrovascular isquémico (ischemic stroke): ahk-see-DEN-teh seh-reh-broh-vas-KOO-lar ees-KEH-mee-koh

3. Epilepsia refractaria (refractory epilepsy): eh-pee-LEP-see-ah reh-frak-TAH-ree-ah

4. Esclerosis múltiple progresiva (progressive multiple sclerosis): es-kleh-ROH-sees MOOL-tee-pleh proh-GREH-see-vah

5. Neuropatía periférica (peripheral neuropathy): ney-roh-pah-TEE-ah peh-ree-FEH-ree-kah

6. Parkinson avanzado (advanced Parkinson's disease): PAR-kin-son ah-vahn-SAH-doh

7. Alzheimer temprano (early-onset Alzheimer's disease): ahl-ZHY-mer tem-PRAH-noh

8. Demencia vascular (vascular dementia): deh-MEN-syah vas-KOO-lar

9. Tumor cerebral maligno (malignant brain tumor): too-MOR seh-reh-BRAL mah-LEEG-noh

10. Parálisis cerebral espástica (spastic cerebral palsy): pah-rah-LEE-sees seh-reh-BRAL es-PAHS-tee-kah

Oftalmología / Ophtalmology

1. Astigmatismo corneal (corneal astigmatism): ah-stee-gma-TEES-mo kor-NEE-ahl

2. Catarata nuclear (nuclear cataract): kah-tah-RAH-tah noo-KLEE-ahr

3. Conjuntivitis alérgica (allergic conjunctivitis): kohn-hoon-tee-VEE-tees ah-LER-hee-kah

4. Glaucoma de ángulo abierto (open-angle glaucoma): glah-OOH-koh-mah deh AHN-goh-loh ah-BYEHR-toh

5. Desprendimiento de retina (retinal detachment): des-pren-dee-MYEN-toh deh reh-TEE-nah

6. Degeneración macular húmeda (wet macular degeneration): deh-heh-nehr-ah-SYON mah-koo-LAR OO-meh-dah

7. Miopía alta (high myopia): mee-oh-PEE-ah AHL-tah

8. Hipermetropía severa (severe hyperopia): ee-per-meh-troh-PEE-ah seh-VEH-rah

9. Queratocono avanzado (advanced keratoconus): keh-rah-toh-KOH-noh ah-vahn-SAH-doh

10. Estrabismo convergente (convergent strabismus): es-trah-BEEZ-moh kon-ver-HEN-the

Dermatología / Dermatology

1. Dermatitis atópica (atopic dermatitis): der-mah-TEE-tees ah-TOH-pee-kah

2. Eczema dishidrótico (dyshidrotic eczema): ehk-SEH-mah dee-see-DROH-tee-koh

3. Melanoma maligno (malignant melanoma): meh-lah-NOH-mah mah-LEEG-noh

4. Psoriasis pustulosa (pustular psoriasis): soh-RYAH-sis poos-too-LOH-sah

5. Acné quístico (cystic acne): ak-NEH KEES-tee-koh

6. Vitíligo segmentario (segmental vitiligo): vee-tee-LEE-goh seg-men-TAH-ree-oh

7. Urticaria crónica (chronic hives): oor-tee-KAH-ree-ah KROH-nee-kah

8. Carcinoma basocelular infiltrante (infiltrating basal cell carcinoma): kar-see-NOH-mah bah-soh-seh-loo-LAR een-feel-TRAN-teh

9. Rosácea eritematotelangiectásica (erythematotelangiectatic rosacea): roh-SAH-seh-ah eh-ree-teh-mah-toh-teh-LAN-jee-ek-TAH-see-kah

10. Herpes zóster oftálmico (ophthalmic shingles): ER-pehs ZOS-tehr off-TAHL-mee-koh

Endocrinología / Endocrinology

1. Diabetes tipo 1 (type 1 diabetes): dee-ah-BEH-tehs TEE-poh oon

2. Tiroiditis de Hashimoto (Hashimoto's thyroiditis): tee-roy-DEET-ees deh hah-shee-MOH-toh

3. Insulinoma pancreático (pancreatic insulinoma): een-soo-lee-NOH-mah pan-kree-ah-TEE-koh

4. Hipotiroidismo congénito (congenital hypothyroidism): ee-poh-tee-roy-DEEZ-moh kon-HEN-ee-toh

5. Hipertiroidismo de Graves (Graves' disease hyperthyroidism): ee-per-tee-roy-DEEZ-moh deh grayvz

6. Enfermedad de Addison (Addison's disease): en-fer-meh-DAHD deh AH-dee-sohn

7. Síndrome de Cushing (Cushing's syndrome): seen-droh-meh deh KOOSH-eeng

8. Resistencia a la insulina (insulin resistance): reh-sees-TEN-syah ah lah een-SOO-lee-nah

9. Hormona del crecimiento (growth hormone): or-MOH-nah del kre-seeh-MYEN-toh

10. Gluconeogénesis (gluconeogenesis): gloo-koh-neh-oh-HEH-neh-sees

Gastroenterología / Gastroenterology

1. Gastroenteritis aguda (acute gastroenteritis): gas-tro-en-teh-REE-tees ah-GOO-dah

2. Úlcera péptica (peptic ulcer): OOL-seh-rah PEP-tee-kah

3. Colitis ulcerativa (ulcerative colitis): koh-LEE-tees ool-seh-rah-TEE-vah

4. Reflujo gastroesofágico (gastroesophageal reflux): reh-FLOO-hoh gas-troh-eh-soh-FAH-hee-koh

5. Hepatitis autoinmune (autoimmune hepatitis): heh-pah-TEE-tees ow-toh-een-MOO-neh

6. Cirrhosis biliar primaria (primary biliary cirrhosis): see-ROH-sees bee-lee-ahr pree-MAHR-ee-ah

7. Pancreatitis necrotizante (necrotizing pancreatitis): pan-kree-ah-TEE-tees neh-kroh-TEE-zahn-teh

8. Enfermedad celíaca (celiac disease): en-fer-meh-DAHD seh-LEE-ah-kah

9. Síndrome del intestino irritable (irritable bowel syndrome): seen-droh-meh del een-tes-TEE-noh eer-ree-TAH-bleh

10. Enfermedad de Crohn (Crohn's disease): en-fer-meh-DAHD deh Krohn

Neumología / Pulmonology

1. Neumonía bacteriana (bacterial pneumonia): new-moh-NEE-ah bak-teh-ree-AH-nah

2. Bronquitis crónica (chronic bronchitis): bron-kee-TEES KROH-nee-kah

3. Enfisema pulmonar (pulmonary emphysema): en-fee-SEH-mah pool-moh-NAR

4. Asma severa (severe asthma): AHS-mah seh-VEH-rah

5. Fibrosis quística (cystic fibrosis): fee-BROH-sees KEES-tee-kah

6. Apnea obstructiva del sueño (obstructive sleep apnea): ap-NEH-ah ob-STRUHK-tee-vah del SWAY-nyoh

7. Tromboembolia pulmonar (pulmonary embolism): trom-boh-em-BOH-lee-ah pool-moh-NAR

8. Hipertensión pulmonar (pulmonary hypertension): ee-per-ten-SYON pool-moh-NAR

9. EPOC exacerbada (exacerbated COPD): EE-poh-kah ek-sah-ser-BAH-dah

10. Silicosis avanzada (advanced silicosis): see-lee-KOH-sees ah-vahn-SAH-dah

Urología / Urology

1. Cistitis intersticial (interstitial cystitis): sis-TYE-tees een-ter-STIH-syal

2. Nefritis lúpica (lupus nephritis): neh-FRY-tees LOO-pee-kah

3. Prostatitis bacteriana (bacterial prostatitis): proh-stuh-TYE-tees bak-teh-ree-AH-nah

4. Litiasis renal recurrente (recurrent kidney stones): lee-TEE-ah-sees reh-NAHL reh-KOOR-ehn-teh

5. Incontinencia urinaria de esfuerzo (stress urinary incontinence): een-kon-tee-NEN-syah oo-ree-NAH-ree-ah deh eh-FWER-zoh

6. Hiperplasia prostática benigna (benign prostatic hyperplasia): ee-per-PLAH-see-ah proh-STAH-tee-kah beh-NEEG-nah

7. Insuficiencia renal crónica (chronic kidney disease): een-soo-fee-SYEN-syah reh-NAHL kroh-NEE-kah

8. Infección urinaria complicada (complicated urinary infection): een-fek-SYON oo-ree-NAH-ree-ah kom-plee-KAH-dah

9. Hematuria persistente (persistent hematuria): heh-mah-TOO-ree-ah per-sis-TEN-teh

10. Disuria obstructiva (obstructive dysuria): dee-SOO-ree-ah ob-STRUHK-tee-vah

Nefrología / Nephrology

1. Insuficiencia renal aguda (acute renal insufficiency): een-soo-fee-SYEN-syah reh-NAHL ah-GOO-dah

2. Nefropatía diabética avanzada (advanced diabetic nephropathy): neh-froh-PAH-thee-ah dye-ah-BET-ee-kah ah-vahn-SAH-dah

3. Síndrome nefrótico primario (primary nephrotic syndrome): neh-FROT-ik seen-DROHM pree-MAHR-ee-oh

4. Glomerulonefritis rápidamente progresiva (rapidly progressive glomerulonephritis): gloh-meh-roo-loh-neh-FRY-tees RAH-pee-dah-men-teh proh-GREH-see-vah

5. Diálisis peritoneal (peritoneal dialysis): dee-AH-lee-sees peh-ree-toh-NEH-ahl

6. Hipertensión renovascular (renovascular hypertension): ee-per-ten-SYON reh-noh-vas-koo-LAR

7. Pielonefritis aguda (acute pyelonephritis): pee-eh-loh-neh-FRY-tees ah-GOO-dah

8. Nefroesclerosis hipertensiva (hypertensive nephrosclerosis): neh-froh-skleh-ROH-sees ee-per-ten-SEE-vah

9. Hiperpotasemia crónica (chronic hyperkalemia): ee-per-poe-tah-SEH-mee-ah kroh-NEE-kah

10. Acidosis tubular renal (renal tubular acidosis): ah-see-DOH-sees too-boo-LAHR reh-NAHL

Infectología / Infectology

1. Sepsis severa (severe sepsis): SEP-sees seh-VEH-rah

2. Meningitis bacteriana (bacterial meningitis): meh-neen-JYE-tees bak-teh-ree-AH-nah

3. Tuberculosis pulmonar (pulmonary tuberculosis): too-ber-kyoo-LOH-sees pool-moh-NAR

4. Hepatitis fulminante (fulminant hepatitis): heh-pah-TEE-tees fool-mee-NAHN-teh

5. Endocarditis infecciosa (infective endocarditis): en-doh-kar-DYE-tees een-fek-SYOH-sah

6. Infección por VIH (HIV infection): een-fek-SYON por VEE-AYH-AH-cheh

7. Leishmaniasis visceral (visceral leishmaniasis): lay-shmah-NYE-ah-sees vee-seh-RAHL

8. Coccidioidomicosis diseminada (disseminated coccidioidomycosis): kohk-see-dee-OY-doh-mee-KOH-sees dee-seh-mee-NAH-dah

9. Criptococosis meníngea (meningeal cryptococcosis): kreep-toh-KOH-koh-sees meh-NEEN-heh-ah

10. Fiebre tifoidea (typhoid fever): fee-EH-breh tee-FOY-deh-ah

Exercise 2: Medical vocabulary practice

To practice your medical vocabulary in Spanish, try the following exercises:

1. Create flashcards with Spanish medical terms on one side and their definitions on the other. Practice regularly until you can quickly and confidently recall the meanings.

2. Read medical texts or articles in Spanish and look up any unfamiliar words.

   Some examples include:

   - "¿Qué es la presión arterial alta?": This article, published by the American Heart Association, provides a straightforward explanation of what blood pressure is, the associated risk factors, and recommended actions for those diagnosed with high blood pressure.

   - " Prevención de enfermedades cardio y cerebrovasculares " is a short article featuring five tips for maintaining good health and preventing diseases. It was published on the Spanish Ministry of Health's website.

   - "Beneficios del ejercicio físico en población sana e impacto sobre la aparición de enfermedad": This article explores the health benefits of physical exercise, offering practical tips for starting out. It was published on Elsevier's website.

3. Listen to Spanish-language medical podcasts, lectures, or webinars to become more familiar with medical terms and their usage. Platforms like Youtube, Spotify, Coursera, and Doc Molly offer ample resources.

4. Practice translating medical terms between English and Spanish to enhance your vocabulary and comprehension of medical terminology in both languages.

Exercise 3: Medical language exchange

Pair up with a native Spanish-speaking healthcare professional for a language exchange. Practice with each other and take turns discussing healthcare topics in both languages. This will allow you to improve your fluency, build your vocabulary, and learn about healthcare practices and culture in Spanish-speaking countries.

Role-playing exercises in diverse medical scenarios

By simulating real-life medical scenarios, you can gain confidence in using medical Spanish terminology and phrases. Below are ten role-playing exercises covering diverse medical scenarios:

Patient history	Conduct a medical interview with a Spanish-speaking patient experiencing stomach pain. Ask the patient about symptoms, including onset and pain location, and gather any other relevant information.
Prescription refills	Discuss prescription refills with a Spanish-speaking patient as a pharmacist. Verify the patient's name and date of birth, ask about any allergies or side effects, and provide medication instructions.
Physical exam	Perform a physical examination on a Spanish-speaking patient. Ask the patient to describe any pain or discomfort, use medical terminology during the examination, and provide instructions for follow-up care.
Emergency room	Treat a Spanish-speaking patient in the emergency room for chest pain. Assess symptoms, take vital signs, and provide emergency treatment.
Pregnancy check-up	Conduct a check-up on a Spanish-speaking pregnant patient. Inquire about symptoms, measure their blood pressure and weight, and provide advice for prenatal care.
Mental health consultation	Consult with a Spanish-speaking patient who is experiencing anxiety. Use medical terminology to explain the diagnosis, offer coping strategies, and recommend treatment options.
Vaccine administration	Administer a vaccine to a Spanish-speaking patient as a nurse. Use medical terminology to explain the purpose of the vaccine, confirm the patient's identity, and provide instructions for follow-up care.
Dental exam	Perform a dental examination on a Spanish-speaking patient. Ask the patient about their dental history, use medical terminology during the exam, and provide follow-up care instructions.

Physical therapy session	Conduct a session with a Spanish-speaking patient recovering from an injury. Use medical terminology to explain the exercises performed as a physical therapist, provide advice for recovery, and recommend follow-up care.
Health education	Provide health education to a Spanish-speaking patient. Use medical terminology to explain the importance of healthy habits, recommend lifestyle changes, and provide resources for additional information.
Confidentiality in teen consultations	Request permission from the mother to speak privately with her daughter to address the teenage patient's sexual health concerns. Explain that it is standard practice to discuss certain topics alone with the patient to ensure comfort and honesty, which is important for providing the best care. Reassure the mother that this is a standard practice and emphasize the importance of confidentiality.

Regional expresions

Spanish is spoken in many countries, and each region has its own unique expressions and slang. Here are some common expressions used in different regions of Latin America:

- Mexico: "Qué onda" – What's up?
- Guatemala: "Pura vida" – Pure life (used to express positivity)
- Colombia: "Chévere" – Cool or great
- Venezuela: "Chamo" – Dude or guy
- Peru: "Chamba" – Work or job
- Argentina: "Boludo" – Stupid or idiot (can also be used affectionately between friends)
- Chile: "Cachai" – Do you understand?
- Ecuador: "Chévere" – Cool or great (similar to Colombia)
- Costa Rica: "Mae" – Dude or guy (similar to Venezuela)
- Cuba: "Qué bola" – What's up?
- Dominican Republic: "Diache" – Wow or oh my god
- Puerto Rico: "Bregar" – To work hard or hustle
- Uruguay: "Laburar" – To work
- Panama: "Sancocho" – A traditional soup made with chicken, plantains, and other ingredients
- Bolivia: "Achachay" – Expression used to express cold or chilliness

- Honduras: "Galillo" – Traditional Honduran dish made with rice, vegetables, and meat
- Nicaragua: "Nica" – Colloquial term for a Nicaraguan person
- El Salvador: "Pupusa" – Traditional Salvadoran dish made with corn masa and filled with cheese, beans, or meat
- Paraguay: "Chipa" – Traditional Paraguayan bread made with manioc flour and cheese
- Brazil: "Saudade" – A feeling of nostalgia or longing for someone or something

By practicing these role-playing exercises, improving your pronunciation, and learning some common expressions used in different regions of Latin America, you can enhance your ability to communicate with Spanish-speaking patients in medical settings. Be mindful to approach patients with cultural sensitivity and respect, and to seek out resources to continue improving your medical Spanish skills.

Cultural competence scenarios

One essential aspect of providing quality healthcare is cultural competence. As a healthcare professional, you must be able to communicate effectively with patients from diverse cultural backgrounds. In this exercise, we will explore some scenarios that highlight the importance of cultural competence.

Scenario 1	As a nurse working in a pediatric clinic, a Spanish-speaking mother brings in her child for a routine check-up. During the examination, you notice a rash on the child's face. The mother tells you that she has been using a traditional home remedy to treat the rash, and the rash has not improved. How would you handle this situation?
	To handle this scenario effectively, you must first acknowledge the mother's concern and show respect for her cultural practices. You can then explain that the rash may require medical treatment and offer to prescribe a medication that is safe and effective for the child's age.
Scenario 2	As a physician assistant working in an urgent care clinic, a Spanish-speaking patient comes in with severe abdominal pain. Family members insist on staying in the exam room during the consultation. How would you handle this situation?
	In this scenario, be sensitive to the patient's cultural values and preferences. Explain that standard practice involves examining the patient in a private room to ensure their comfort and confidentiality. You can offer to provide an interpreter if necessary to ensure that the patient's concerns are fully understood.

Scenario 3	As a physical therapist working with a Spanish-speaking patient who has recently immigrated to the United States, you notice that the patient is hesitant to participate in the therapy exercises and seems uncomfortable. How would you handle this situation?
	Recognize the potential cultural barriers that may be impacting the patient's comfort and participation in therapy. Start by acknowledging the patient's cultural background and asking if there are any cultural practices that you should be aware of. Explain the importance of the therapy exercises and offer to modify the exercises to better suit the patient's needs and preferences. Additionally, consider enlisting the help of a cultural liaison or interpreter to facilitate communication and ensure that the patient is comfortable and engaged in the therapy process.

Vocabulary review games

Vocabulary review games can be a fun and engaging way to practice medical terminology in Spanish. Here are a few games that you can try:

Game 1	Flashcard Relay	Divide into teams and create flashcards with medical terms in Spanish on one side and their English translations on the other. The first team member runs to the board and picks up a flashcard, reads the Spanish term aloud, and then passes the card to the next team member, who reads the English translation. The first team to finish the relay wins.
Game 2	Medical Bingo	Create bingo cards with medical terms in Spanish on each square. Call out the English translations, and players must mark off the corresponding square on their bingo card. The first player to get bingo wins.
Game 3	Medical Pictionary	Divide into teams and have one team member draw a medical term in Spanish while the other team members try to guess the term. The first team to guess correctly wins a point. Rotate roles so that each team member gets a chance to draw.

Listening comprehension

Listening comprehension is an important skill in medical Spanish. In this exercise, you will listen to audio recordings of medical conversations or lectures in Spanish and answer questions about what you heard. You can find resources online, such as Spanish-language medical podcasts or lectures, or create your own recordings.

Here are a few examples of questions you could ask:

1. What is the patient's main complaint?

2. What medications is the patient taking?

3. What is the diagnosis?

4. What treatment options are being discussed?

5. What is the patient's prognosis?

This exercise will help you improve your ability to understand spoken medical Spanish, which is especially important when communicating with patients who may not be fluent in English.

Conclusion

In this chapter, we explored additional practice exercises that will help you improve your medical Spanish skills. Cultural competence scenarios, vocabulary review games, and listening comprehension exercises will challenge you to apply your knowledge in different contexts, reinforce your vocabulary, and improve your listening comprehension. Remember to practice regularly, immerse yourself in Spanish-language healthcare contexts, and seek opportunities to speak with native Spanish speakers to continue improving your skills. With dedication and persistence, you will be able to speak medical Spanish confidently and effectively in no time!

Chapter 5:
Appendices

The patient is the most important person in the hospital.

Sister Mary Jean Dorcy

This chapter offers healthcare professionals a valuable set of appendices to aid in their efforts in learning medical Spanish. The appendices contain a variety of resources such as a list of medical abbreviations in Spanish, a glossary of medical Spanish terms, conjugations and pronunciation guides, and a comprehensive Spanish-English and English-Spanish medical dictionary.

Medical abbreviations in Spanish

In the medical field, abbreviations are commonly used to save time and space. However, it is important to note that not all medical abbreviations in Spanish have the same meaning as their English counterparts. Here are 50 commonly used medical abbreviations in Spanish:

Abbreviation	Spanish meaning	English meaning
AC	Antes de comer	Before eating
BH	Biometría hemática/ Hemograma completo	Complete blood count
CC	Centrímetros Cubícos	Cubic centimeters
EKG	Electrocargiograma	Electrocardiogram
IM	Intramuscular	Intramuscular
IVU	Infección de las vías urinarias / Infección del tracto urinario	Urinary tract infection
IV	Intravenoso	Intravenously
PA or TA	Presión arterial	Blood pressure
Rx	Rayos X	X Rays
Px	Paciente	Patient
SNG	Sonda nasogástrica	Nasogastric tube

Abbreviation	Spanish meaning	English meaning
TB	Tuberculosis	Tuberculosis
TBC	Test de tuberculina	Tuberculin test
TPR	Temperatura, pulso, respiración	Temperature, pulse, respiration
UCI	Unidad de cuidados intensivos	Intensive care unit
UCIN	Unidad de Cuidados Intensivos Neonatales	Neonatal Intensive Care Unit
URO	Urología	Urology
VHC	Virus de la hepatitis C	Hepatitis C virus
VO	Vía oral	Orally
VS	Vía subcutánea	Subcutaneously
VHB	Virus de la hepatitis B	Hepatitis B virus
VIH	Virus de la inmunodeficiencia humana	Human immunodeficiency virus
OMS	Organización Mundial de la Salud	World Health Organization
TC	Tomografía computarizada	Computed tomography
RM	Resonancia magnética	Magnetic resonance
EEG	Electroencefalograma	Electroencephalogram
TO	Terapia ocupacional	Occupational therapy
TH	Terapia del habla	Speech therapy
TF	Terapia física	Physical therapy
AAS	Ácido acetilsalicílico	Acetylsalicylic acid
AB	Aborto	Abortion
ACTH	Hormona adrenocorticótropa	Adrenocorticotropic hormone
AGA	Adecuado para la edad gestacional	Adequate for gestational age
ALT	Alanina aminotransferasa	Alanine aminotransferase
AST	Aspartato aminotransferasa	Aspartate aminotransferase
BCG	Bacilo de Calmette y Guérin	Bacillus of Calmette and Guérin
BPD	Displasia broncopulmonar	Bronchopulmonary dysplasia
EPOC	Enfermedad Pulmonar Obstructiva Crónica	Chronic Obstructive Pulmonary Disease
GGT	Gamma glutamil transferasa	Gamma glutamyl transferase

Abbreviation	Spanish meaning	English meaning
Hb	Hemoglobina	Hemoglobin
hCG	Gonadotropina coriónica humana	Human chorionic gonadotropin
HTA	Hipertensión arterial	Arterial hypertension
DM	Diabetes mellitus	Diabetes mellitus
PCR	Reacción en cadena de la polimerasa	Polymerase Chain Reaction
PTH	Hormona paratiroidea	Parathyroid hormone
TSH	Hormona estimulante de la tiroides	Thyroid-stimulating hormone

Glossary of medical Spanish terms

In this glossary, we have compiled a list of all the medical Spanish terms covered in this book, along with their corresponding English translations.

Spanish	English
Corazón	Heart
Riñón	Kidney
Pulmón	Lung
Hígado	Liver
Cerebro	Brain
Sangre	Blood
Hueso	Bone
Cáncer	Cancer
Infección	Infection
Diabetes	Diabetes
Enfermedad	Disease
Fiebre	Fever
Dolor	Pain
Presión arterial	Blood pressure
Vacuna	Vaccine
Tratamiento	Treatment
Antibiótico	Antibiotic

Spanish	English
Inflamación	Inflammation
Radiografía	X-ray
Nutrición	Nutrition
Paciente	Patient
Terapia	Therapy
Síntomas	Symptoms
Salud	Health
Cirugía	Surgery
Dosis	Dose
Medicamento	Medication
Venas	Veins
Músculo	Muscle
Hormona	Hormone
Terapeuta	Therapist
Especialista	Specialist
Epidemia	Epidemic
Contagio	Contagion
Medicina	Medicine
Órganos	Organs
Enfermera	Nurse
Deshidratación	Dehydration
Asma	Asthma
Infarto	Heart attack
Anestesia	Anesthesia
Trasplante	Transplant
Hemorragia	Hemorrhage
Psiquiatría	Psychiatry
Traumatismo	Trauma
Síndrome	Syndrome
Virus	Virus

Spanish	English
Quimioterapia	Chemotherapy
Radioterapia	Radiation therapy
Human body systems and apparatuses	
Sistema circulatorio	Circulatory system
Sistema digestivo	Digestive system
Sistema endocrino	Endocrine system
Sistema inmunológico	Immune system
Sistema nervioso	Nervous system
Sistema respiratorio	Respiratory system
Sistema urinario	Urinary system
Prescription and Medication	
Antibiótico	Antibiotic
Antiinflamatorio	Anti-inflammatory
Analgésico	Pain reliever
Antihipertensivos	Antihypertensive drug
Insulina	Insulin
Esteroides	Steroids
Vacuna	Vaccine
Antidepresivo	Antidepressant
Rx Medication	
Prescription and Medication	
Amoxicilina	Amoxicilin
Cefalexina	Cephalexin
Paracetamol (Acetaminofén)	Paracetamol (Acetaminophen)
Ibuprofeno	Ibuprofen
Diazepam	Diazepam
Omeprazol	Omeprazole
Enalapril	Enalapril
Metformina	Metformin
Simvastatina	Simvastatin

Prescription and Medication

Insulina	Insulin
Prednisona	Prednisone
Furosemida	Furosemide
Alprazolam	Alprazolam
Ranitidina	Ranitidine
Atorvastatina	Atorvastatin
Losartán	Losartan
Amoxicilina con ácido clavulánico	Amoxicillin with Clavulanic Acid
Metoprolol	Metoprolol
Clonazepam	Clonazepam
Levotiroxina	Levothyroxine

OTC medication

Aspirina	Aspirin
Loratadina	Loratadine
Ranitidina	Ranitidine
Naproxeno	Naproxen
Antiácidos	Antiacids
Vitamina C	Vitamin C
Dextrometorfano	Dextromethorphan
Salbutamol	Salbutamol
Ibuprofeno con pseudoefedrina	Ibuprofen with Pseudoephedrine
Ketoprofeno	Ketoprofen
Paracetamol con pseudoefedrina	Paracetamol with Pseudoephedrine
Acetaminofén con codeína	Acetaminophen with Codeine
Clorfeniramina	Chlorpheniramine
Loperamida	Loperamide
Lansoprazol	Lansoprazole
Metamizol	Metamizole
Magnesio	Magnesium

Clinical and imaging studies	
Tomografía computarizada	CT scan
Radiografía	X-ray
Resonancia magnética	MRI
Electrocardiograma	ECG
Examen de sangre	Blood test
Examen de orina / urianalisis	Urine test
Examen de heces	Stool test
Endoscopía	Endoscopy
Colonoscopía	Colonoscopy
Biopsia	Biopsy
Cirugía	Surgery
Anestesia	Anesthesia
Terapia física	Physical therapy
Terapia ocupacional	Occupational therapy
Terapia del habla	Speech therapy
Terapia respiratoria	Respiratory therapy
Hemodiálisis	Hemodialysis
Quimioterapia	Chemotherapy
Radioterapia	Radiation therapy
Trasplante	Transplant
Tacto rectal	Rectal examination
Antígeno prostático	Prostatic antigen

	Diet	
MEXICO	Tacos	Tacos
	Pozole	Pozole
	Tamales	Tamales
	Quesadillas	Quesadillas

HONDURAS	Baleadas	Baleadas
	Sopa de caracol	Snail soup
	Sopa de pescado seco	Dry fish soup
	Atol de elote	Corn atoll
GUATEMA-LA	Pepian	Pepian (a traditional Guatemalan stew)
	Kak'ik	Kak'ik (a traditional Guatemalan turkey soup)
	Plátanos en mole	Plantains in mole sauce
	Tamales colorados	Colored tamales
ARGENTINA	Asado	Argentine barbecue
	Empanadas	Stuffed pastry turnovers
	Milanesas	Breaded and fried meat cutlet
	Chimichurri	Traditional Argentine herb sauce
	Provoleta	Grilled provolone cheese
COLOMBIA	Bandeja paisa	Paisa
	Ajiaco	Chicken and potato soup
	Arepas	Cornmeal cakes
	Sancocho	Traditional stew
	Lechona	Roasted pig stuffed with rice and peas
CUBA	Ropa vieja	Shredded beef stew
	Lechón asado	Roast pork
	Picadillo	Ground beef hash
	Tostones	Fried green plantains
		Black beans and rice

Conjugations and pronunciation guides

To effectively engage with Spanish-speaking patients, healthcare professionals need a strong grasp of verb conjugations and precise pronunciation. Review these 20 examples of verb conjugations and pronunciation to improve your communication skills:

Hablar (to speak)

Yo hablo	I speak
Tú hablas	You speak
Él/ella habla	He/she speaks
Nosotros/as hablamos	We speak
Ellos/ellas hablan	They speak
Ustedes hablan	You all speak

Pronunciation: ah-blahr

Escuchar (to listen)

Yo escucho	I listen
Tú escuchas	You listen
Él/ella escucha	He/she listens
Nosotros/as escuchamos	We listen
Ustedes escuchan	You all listen
Ellos/ellas escuchan	They listen

Pronunciation: ess-koo-char

Preguntar (to ask)

Yo pregunto	I ask
Tú preguntas	You ask
Él/ella pregunta	He/she asks
Nosotros/as preguntamos	We ask
Ustedes preguntan	You all ask
Ellos/ellas preguntan	They ask

Pronunciation: preh-goon-tahr

Explicar (to explain)

Yo explico	I explain
Tú explicas	You explain

Explicar (to explain)

Él/ella explica	He/she explains
Nosotros/as explicamos	We explain
Ustedes explican	You all explain
Ellos/ellas explican	They explain

Pronunciation: ess-plee-kahr

Comprender (to understand)

Yo comprendo	I understand
Tú comprendes	You understand
Él/ella comprende	He/she understands
Nosotros/as comprendemos	We understand
Ustedes comprenden	You all understand
Ellos/ellas comprenden	They understand

Pronunciation: kohm-prehn-dehr

Decir (to say)

Yo digo	I say
Tú dices	You say
Él/ella dice	He/she says
Nosotros/as decimos	We say
Ustedes dicen	You all say
Ellos/ellas dicen	They say

Pronunciation: deh-seer

Hacer (to do/make)

Yo hago	I do/make
Tú haces	(You do/make)
Él/ella hace	He/she does/makes
Nosotros/as hacemos	We do/make

Hacer (to do/make)

Ustedes hacen	You all do/make
Ellos/ellas hacen	They do/make

Pronunciation: ah-sehr

Tomar (to take)

Yo tomo	I take
Tú tomas	You take
Él/ella toma	He/she takes
Nosotros/as tomamos	We take
Ustedes toman	You all take
Ellos/ellas toman	They take

Pronunciation: toh-mahr

Cuidar (to care for)

Yo cuido	I care for
Tú cuidas	You care for
Él/ella cuida	He/she cares for
Nosotros/as cuidamos	We care for
Ustedes cuidan	You all care for
Ellos/ellas cuidan	They care for

Pronunciation: kwee-dahr

Ayudar (to help)

Yo ayudo	I help
Tú ayudas	You help
Él/ella ayuda	He/she helps
Nosotros/as ayudamos	We help
Ustedes ayudan	You all help
Ellos/ellas ayudan	They help

Pronunciation: ah-yoo-dahr

Examinar (to examine)

Yo examino	I examine
Tú examinas	You examine
Él/ella examina	He/she examines
Nosotros/as examinamos	We examine
Ustedes examinan	You all examine
Ellos/ellas examinan	They examine

Pronunciation: eks-sah-mee-nahr

Tratar (to treat)

Yo trato	I treat
Tú tratas	You treat
Él/ella trata	He/she treats
Nosotros/as tratamos	We treat
Ustedes tratan	You all treat
Ellos/ellas tratan	They treat

Pronunciation: trah-tahr

Recetar (to prescribe)

Yo receto	I prescribe
Tú recetas	You prescribe
Él/ella receta	He/she prescribes
Nosotros/as recetamos	We prescribe
Ustedes recetan	You all prescribe
Ellos/ellas recetan	They prescribe

Pronunciation: reh-seh-tahr

Curar (to cure)

Yo curo	I cure
Tú curas	You cure
Él/ella cura	He/she cures

Curar (to cure)	
Nosotros/as curamos	We cure
Usteden curan	You all cure
Ellos/ellas curan	They cure
Pronunciation: koo-rahr	

Diagnosticar (to diagnose)	
Yo diagnostic	I diagnose
Tú diagnosticas	You diagnose
Él/ella diagnostica	He/she diagnoses
Nosotros/as diagnosticamos	We diagnose
Ustedes diagnostican	You all diagnose
Ellos/ellas diagnostican	They diagnose
Pronunciation: dee-ahg-nos-tee-kahr	

Monitorear (to monitor)	
Yo monitoreo	I monitor
Tú monitoreas	You monitor
Él/ella monitorea	He/she monitors
Nosotros/as monitoreamos	We monitor
Usteden monitorean	You all monitor
Ellos/ellas monitorean	They monitor
Pronunciation: moh-nee-toh-reh-ahr	

Prevenir (to prevent)	
Yo prevengo	I prevent
Tú previenes	You prevent
Él/ella previene	He/she prevents
Nosotros/as prevenimos	We prevent
Ustedes previenen	You all prevent

Prevenir (to prevent)

Ellos/ellas previenen	They prevent

Pronunciation: preh-veh-neer

Desinfectar (to disinfect)

Yo desinfecto	I disinfect
Tú desinfectas	You disinfect
Él/ella desinfecta	He/she disinfects
Nosotros/as desinfectamos	We disinfect
Ustedes desinfectan	You all disinfect
Ellos/ellas desinfectan	They disinfect

Pronunciation: deh-seen-fehk-tahr

Operar (to operate)

Yo opero	I operate
Tú operas	You operate
Él/ella opera	He/she operates
Nosotros/as operamos	We operate
Ustedes operan	You all operate
Ellos/ellas operan	They operate

Pronunciation: oh-peh-rahr

Vacunar (vaccinate)

Yo vacuno	I vaccinate
Tú vacunas	You vaccinate
Él/ella vacuna	He/she vaccinates
Nosotros/as vacunamos	We vaccinate
Ustedes vacunan	You vaccinate
Ellos/ellas vacunan	They vaccinate

Pronunciation: bah-koo-nahr

Spanish-English and English-Spanish medical dictionary

A medical dictionary can be a valuable resource to help healthcare professionals bridge language barriers Spanish-speaking patients. Below are some examples of medical terms paired with their translations:

A	
Abdomen	Abdomen
Aborto	Abortion
Absceso	Abscess
Acné	Acne
Agudo	Acute
Adicción	Addiction
Alergia	Allergy
Ambulancia	Ambulance
Anemia	Anemia
Anestesia	Anesthesia
Aneurisma	Aneurysm
Anorexia	Anorexia
Antibiótico	Antibiotic
Ansiedad	Anxiety
Arritmia	Arrhytmia
Atrofia	Atrophy
Avulsión	Avulsion
Adrenérgico	Adrenergic
Afasia	Aphasia
Ateroesclerosis	Atherosclerosis
B	
Bacteria	Bacteria
Bazo	Spleen
Biopsia	Biopsy
Bronquitis	Bronchitis

Boca	Mouth
Brazo	Arm
Bulto	Lump
Bebé	Baby
Billirubina	Bilirubin
Benigno	Benign
Bocio	Goiter
Bacteremia	Bacteremia
Brote	Outbreak
Bilis	Bile
Bolo alimenticio	Food bolus

C

Cabeza	Head
Cáncer	Cancer
Células	Cells
Corazón	Heart
Cerebro	Brain
Cirugía	Surgery
Columna vertebral	Spine
Cuerpo	Body
Cicatriz	Scar
Cáncer de mama	Breast cancer
Cáncer de próstata	Prostate cáncer
Colecistitis	Cholecystitis
Catarata	Cataract
Cálculo	Stone
Cápsula	Capsule

D

Dolor	Pain
Dedo	Finger

Diente	Tooth
Diarrea	Diarrhea
Depresión	Depression
Digestión	Digestion
Dermatitis	Dermatitis
Dolor de cabeza	Headache
Dolor de espalda	Back pain
Dolor abdominal	Abdominal pain
Desidratación	Dehydration
Dismenorrea	Dysmenorrhea
Displasia	Dysplasia
Dolor torácico	Chest pain
E	
Enfermedad	Illness
Estómago	Stomach
Espalda	Back
Esófago	Esophagus
Enfermedad cardiovascular	Cardiovascular disease
Enfermedad respiratoria	Respiratory disease
Enfermedad infecciosa	Infectious disease
Epidemia	Epidemic
Enfermedad crónica	Chronic disease
Edema	Edema
Encefalitis	Encephalitis
Enfermedad renal	Kidney disease
Eritema	Erythema
Esclerosis multiple	Multiple sclerosis
F	
Fiebre	Fever
Fractura	Fracture

Flema	Phlegm
Fatiga	Fatigue
Faringitis	Pharyngitis
Fosas nasales	Nasal cavities
Feto	Fetus
Fibrilación auricular	Atrial fibrillation
Fibroma	Fibroma
Fibrosis	Fibrosis
Fístula	Fistula
Fisioterapia	Physiotherapy
Flatulencia	Flatulence
Flujo vaginal	Vaginal discharge
Fascitis	Fasciitis
G	
Garganta	Throat
Gripe	Flu
Gangrena	Gangrene
Gastroenteritis	Gastroenteritis
Ginecología	Gynecology
Genitales	Genitals
Glaucoma	Glaucoma
Gingivitis	Gingivitis
Gonorrea	Gonorrhea
Granuloma	Granuloma
Glándula	Gland
Glóbulo rojo	Red blood cell
Gota	Gout
H	
Hígado	Liver
Herida	Wound

Hipertensión	Hypertension
Hemorragia	Hemorrhage
Hueso	Bone
Hueso fracturado	Fractured brone
Hemofilia	Hemophilia
Hiperactividad	Hyperactivity
Hipercolesterolemia	Hypercholesterolemia
Hipertermia	Hypertermia
Hematoma	Hematoma
Hidratación	Hydration
Hidrocefalia	Hydrocephalus
Hiperplasia	Hyperplasia
Hipoglucemia	Hypoglucemia
I	
Infección	Infection
Immunidad	Immunity
Inflamación	Inflammation
Influenza	Influenza
Insuficiencia cardíaca	Heart failure
Insulina	Insulin
Ictericia	Jaundice
Inyección	Injection
Isquemia	Ischemia
Infarto	Infarction
Incontinencia urinaria	Urinary incontinence
Insuficiencia renal	Renal insufficiency
Intoxicación	Intoxication
Íleo	Ileus
Impétigo	impetigo
J	

Jeringa	Syringe
Jugo gástrico	Gastric juice
Joroba	Hump
Jarabe	Syrup
Juanete (hallux valgus)	Bunion (hallux valgus)
Jugo gástrico	Gastric secretion
K	
Kinesioterapia	Kinesiotherapy
Kilcaloría	Kilocalorie
Ketonemia	Ketonemia
Ketosis	Ketosis
Kinasa	Kinasa
Ketonuria	Ketonuria
L	
Laringe	Larynx
Líquido cefalorraquídeo	Cerebrospinal fluid
Llaga	Sore
Laringitis	Laryngitis
Lengua	Tongue
Lesión	Injury
Linfoma	Lymphoma
Linfoadenopatía	Lymphadenopathy
M	
Médico	Physician
Mujer	Woman
Músculo	Muscle
Muela	Tooth
Molestia	Discomfort
Mareo	Dizziness
Muela del juicio	Wisdom tooth

Melanoma	Melanoma
Miastenia	Myasthenia
Miocardio	Myocardium
Miopía	Myopia
N	
Nariz	Nose
Neumonía	Pneumonia
Nervio	Nerve
Naúsea	Nausea
Necrosis	Necrosis
Neuritis	Neuritis
Necrotizante	Necrotizing
Nódulo	Nodule
Nefritis	Nephritis
Neoplasia	Neoplasia
Narcolepsia	Narcolepsy
O	
Oído	Ear
Osteoporosis	Osteoporosis
Ovario	Ovary
Orina	Urina
Odontología	Dentistry
Oftalmología	Ophthalmology
Ortopedia	Orthopedics
Oclusión	Occlusion
Onicomicosis	Onychomycosis
Orzuelo	Sty
Ortopédico	Orthopedic
Otitis	Otitis
P	

Pulmón	Lung
Presión arterial	Blood pressure
Piel	Skin
Parto	Delivery
Páncreas	Pancreas
Parálisis	Paralysis
Parkinson	Parkinson
Pus	Pus
Pericardio	Pericardium
Pancreatitis	Pancreatitis
Poliomielitis	Poliomyelitis
Poliuria	Polyuria
Pseudomonas	Pseudomonas
Psoriasis	Psoriasis
Q	
Quimioterapia	Chemotherapy
Quiste	Cyst
Quemadura	Burn
Queratitis	Keratitis
Quilotórax	Chylothorax
Quilotripsina	Chymotrypsin
Quiluria	Chyluria
Quimioembolización	Chemoembolization
R	
Riñón	Kidney
Reflujo	Reflux
Rinitis	Rhinitis
Resfriado	Cold
Retina	Retina
Reumatismo	Rheumatism

Ronquido	Snore
Rubeola	Rubella
Rabia	Rabies
Rectorragia	Rectal bleeding
Retinopatía	Retinopathy
Ruptura	Rupture
Ruptura prematura de membranas	Premature rupture of membranes
Riesgo cardiovascular	Cardiovascular risk
Radioterapia	Radiation therapy
S	
Sangre	Blood
Síndrome	Syndrome
Sistema nervioso	Nervous system
Sudor	Sweat
Sífilis	Syphilis
Sarampión	Measles
Síndrome de Down	Down syndrome
Sistema inmunológico	Immune system
Sobrepeso	Overweight
Sordera	Deafness
Síndrome metabólico	Metabolic syndrome
T	
Tiroides	Thyroid
Tumor	Tumor
Tratamiento	Treatment
Tuberculosis	Tuberculosis
Terapia	Therapy
Tos	Cough
Trasplante	Transplante
Trombosis	Thrombosis

Triglicéridos	Tryglicerides
Tétanos	Tetanus
Trastorno	Disorder
Trombocitopenia	Thrombocytopenia
Tiroiditis	Thyroiditis
U	
Uretra	Urethra
Urticaria	Urticaria
Úlcera	Ulcer
Uña	Nail
Ultrasonido	Ultrasound
Urgencia	Emergency
Uveítis	Uveitis
Uremia	Uremia
Uropatía	Uropathy
Urolitiasis	Urolithiasis
Úlcera gástrica	Gastric ulcer
V	
Vena	Vein
Vacuna	Vaccine
Varicela	Chickenpox
Vesícula	Vesicle
Vómito	Vomit
Virus	Virus
Vértebra	Vertebra
Várices	Varicose Veins
Vesícula biliar	Gallbladder
Vértigo	Vertigo
Vasculitis	Vasculitis
Venopunción	Venipuncture

Vía intravenosa	Intravenous route
Vasoconstricción	Vasoconstriction
X	
Xantomas	Xanthomas
Xerodermia pigmentosa	Xeroderma pigmentosum
Xeroftalmia	Xerophthalmia
Xerostomía	Xerostomia
Xenotrasplante	Xenotransplantation
Xerosis	Xerosis
Xantelasma	Xanthelasma
Xantinuria	Xanthinuria
Y	
Yodo	Iodine
Yersinia	Yersinia
Yeyuno	Jejunum
Yodo radioactivo	Radioactive iodine
Yeso	Plaster
Yunque	Anvil
Z	
Zóster	Zoster
Zinc	Zinc
Zoonosis	Zoonosis
Zoofilia	Zoophilia
Zoonótico	Zoonotic
Zumbido en los oidos	Ringing in the ears
Zonza pelúcida	Zona pellucida

Chapter VI: Conclusion

The physician's highest calling, his only calling, is to make sick people healthy— to heal, as it is termed.

Samuel Hahnemann

Book structure

Diving the book into three distinct volumes holds immense significance for several reasons. First, it allows for a more focused and organized approach to covering the vast topic of Medical Spanish. Each book can be tailored to address specific aspects of the subject, ensuring a comprehensive yet manageable learning experience for the readers.

Book 1 serves as a foundational introduction, providing readers to the basics of Medical Spanish and language learning techniques. Covering fundamental topics such as the alphabet, medical terminology, and pronunciation, learners can build a strong linguistic groundwork. Additionally, the suggested study plan provides a clear roadmap for achieving fluency within a reasonable timeframe.

Book 2 expands on the linguistic foundation by exploring deeper into medical communication. Structured into sections dedicated to anatomy, medical procedures, prescriptions and emergencies, it allows for a focused examination of important medical contexts. This approach enables healthcare professionals to gain a nuanced understanding of the language used in specific healthcare scenarios, thus enhancing their ability to communicate effectively with patients.

Book 3 focuses on cultural competence, recognizing the importance of understanding the cultural context in healthcare interactions. It provides valuable insights into the cultural diversity within the Spanish-speaking community and offers practical guidance on effective communication strategies. By addressing cultural concepts and practices specific to Hispanic healthcare, this book equips healthcare professionals with the necessary knowledge to provide personalized, compassionate, and culturally competent care.

Dividing the book into three volumes enables readers to navigate the content systematically, progressively enhancing their language skills and cultural awareness. It allows for more flexibility in learning, enabling learners to focus on specific areas of interest or to revisit certain topics for reinforcement. Moreover, the division makes the content more accessible to both beginners and those seeking to deepen their understanding of Medical Spanish and cultural competence in healthcare.

Book highlights

Throughout the book, we achieved significant milestones, starting with the basics of the Spanish language, progressing to medical terminology, and culminating in cultural competence in healthcare. Practical examples and exercises are integrated throughout the book, allowing readers to apply their knowledge in real-world situations.

- In the Spanish Basics section, we covered the Spanish alphabet, sounds, vowels, and consonants, with useful phrases for greetings and introductions, and we emphasized the importance of consistent practice and immersion in the language.

- In the Basic Medical Terminology section, we introduced medical terminology, common medical terms and phrases in Spanish, and pronunciation and spelling rules for medical Spanish.

- In the Anatomy and Physiology section, we explored basic anatomy and physiology terms in Spanish, parts of the body and their functions, and medical conditions and diseases related to the body systems.

- In the Medical Procedures and Exams section, we provided vocabulary for medical procedures and exams in Spanish, common questions and phrases for patient consultations, and how to give instructions to patients in Spanish.

- In the Prescription and Medication section, we covered Spanish terms for prescription and medication, how to inquire about allergies and side effects in Spanish. We also highlighted common R.X. and OTC medications in Spanish.

- In the Medical Emergencies section, we focused on vocabulary and phrases for emergency situations, how to give directions to first responders in Spanish, and how to communicate with patients during an emergency in Spanish.

- Throughout all chapters, we included examples of conversations between healthcare professionals and patients to demonstrate how medical terminology is used in real-life situations.

- In the Enhancing Cultural Competence in Healthcare section, we addressed cultural diversity in healthcare, strategies for delivering culturally competent care for Spanish-speaking patients, effective communication approached, understanding common patient responses, and the Spanish naming system. Real-life conversations demonstrated how cultural competence enhances patient outcomes.

- In the Cultural Concepts in Hispanic Healthcare section, we explored topics such as building trust, traditional healing practices, understanding common ailments, navigating formal and informal healthcare settings within the Hispanic community, the role of Hispanics in the U.S., defining Hispanic or Latino identity, and the importance of the Latino family in healthcare. Conversations between healthcare professionals and patients illustrated the impact of cultural competence on patient care.

- In the Additional Practice Exercises section, we provided role-playing exercises for diverse medical scenarios to reinforce learning and boost confidence when communicating with Spanish-speaking patients. We also included guidance of confidently pronouncing Spanish words and regional expressions.

- In the Appendices, we compiled resources including medical abbreviations in Spanish, a glossary of medical Spanish terms, conjugation and pronunciation guides, and a Spanish-English and English-Spanish medical dictionary.

Book conclusion

Congratulations on completing "Learn Medical Spanish for Healthcare Professionals: Essential Medical Terminology, Words, and Phrases Made Easy"! We trust that this book has been a valuable resource in your journey to become a more effective healthcare provider.

In today's diverse healthcare landscape, effective communication with patients of various cultures and languages is crucial for doctors, nurses, and hospital staff. By learning medical Spanish, you can bridge the language barrier and provide high-quality care to Hispanic patients.

Not only does learning medical Spanish improve patient clinical outcomes, but it also reduces medical errors and increases patient satisfaction. As a healthcare professional, being able to communicate with your patients is essential to building trust and rapport.

This book covers very valuable material, including medical terminology, anatomy and physiology, medical procedures and exams, prescription and medication details, handling medical emergencies, cultural competence in healthcare, insights into Hispanic healthcare concepts, and additional practice exercises. It's a comprehensive guide that equips healthcare professionals with the knowledge and skills necessary to communicate effectively with Spanish-speaking patients.

It's important to remember that mastering medical Spanish goes beyond memorizing terms; it involves understanding the cultural contexts in which these terms are used. Cultural awareness allows you to provide more sensitive and personalized care.

We encourage you to continue practicing your medical Spanish skills in real-life situations. Consider shadowing bilingual colleagues, volunteering at community health centers, provide high-quality care to Hispanic immigrants from less favored sources or practice with a language exchange partner. By actively using the language, you will continuously improve your skills and provide better care to your patients.

In conclusion, we hope that this book has inspired you to embark on a lifelong journey of language and cultural learning. Armed with these tools and knowledge, we trust you'll make a profound difference in the lives of your Spanish-speaking patients. Thank you for choosing "Learn Medical Spanish for Healthcare Professionals: Essential Medical Terminology, Words, and Phrases Made Easy." We wish you continued success in your language-learning journey and in providing high-quality care to a diverse patient population.

Bibliography

1. Lopez, M. H., & Gonzalez-Barrera, A. (2020, July 27). What is the future of Spanish in the United States? Pew Research Center. https://www.pewresearch.org/fact-tank/2013/09/05/what-is-the-future-of-spanish-in-the-united-states/

2. Diez, M. S. (2022, July 21). By 2050, the U.S. could have more Spanish speakers than any other country. Quartz. https://qz.com/441174/by-2050-united-states-will-have-more-spanish-speakers-than-any-other-country

3. U.S. Census Bureau. (2021, October 8). Hispanic Population to Reach 111 Million by 2060. Census.gov. https://www.census.gov/library/visualizations/2018/comm/hispanic-projected-pop.html

4. Proctor, K., Wilson-Frederick, S. M., & Haffer, S. C. (2017). The Limited English Proficient Population: Describing Medicare, Medicaid, and Dual Beneficiaries. Health Equity, 2(1), 82-89. https://doi.org/10.1089/heq.2017.0036

5. Statista. (2024, May 22). Hispanic population in the U.S. 2022, by origin. https://www.statista.com/statistics/234852/us-hispanic-population/

6. Paredes, A. Z., Idrees, J. J., Beal, E. W., Chen, Q., Cerier, E., Okunrintemi, V., Olsen, G., Sun, S., Cloyd, J. M., & Pawlik, T. M. (2018). Influence of English proficiency on patient-provider communication and shared decision-making. Surgery, 163(6), 1220–1225. https://doi.org/10.1016/j.surg.2018.01.012

7. Kim, G., Worley, C. B., Allen, R. S., Vinson, L., Crowther, M. R., Parmelee, P., & Chiriboga, D. A. (2011). Vulnerability of older Latino and Asian immigrants with limited English proficiency. Journal of the American Geriatrics Society, 59(7), 1246–1252. https://doi.org/10.1111/j.1532-5415.2011.03483.x

8. Shamsi, H. A., Almutairi, A. G., Mashrafi, S. A., & Kalbani, T. A. (2020). Implications of Language Barriers for Healthcare: A Systematic Review. Oman Medical Journal, 35(2), e122. https://doi.org/10.5001/omj.2020.40

9. Breaking Down Language Barriers: The Essential Role of Bilingual Nurses. (2021, 17 diciembre). https://www.stkate.edu/academics/healthcare-degrees/breaking-down-language-barriers-essential-role-bilingual-nurses

10. McCarthy, M., Barry, K., Estrada, C., Veliz, B., Rosales, D., Leonard, M., & De Groot, A. S. (2021). Recruitment, Training, and Roles of the Bilingual, Bicultural Navegantes: Developing a Specialized Workforce of Community Health Workers to Serve a Low-Income, Spanish-Speaking Population in Rhode Island. Frontiers in public health, 9, 666566. https://doi.org/10.3389/fpubh.2021.666566

11. Exclusión de «ch» y «ll» del abecedario. (s. f.). Real Acdemia Española. Retrieved April 11 of 2023, from https://www.rae.es/espanol-al-dia/exclusion-de-ch-y-ll-del-abecedario

12. Real Academia Española. (2005). Representación de sonidos. Diccionario panhispánico de dudas. Retrieved April 11th of 2023, from https://www.rae.es/dpd/ayuda/representacion-de-sonidos

13. REAL ACADEMIA ESPAÑOLA: Diccionario de la lengua española, 23.ª ed., [versión 23.6 en línea]. <https://dle.rae.es> Retrieved April 11th of 2023

14. Karliner, L. S., Napoles-Springer, A. M., Schillinger, D., Bibbins-Domingo, K., & Pérez-Stable, E. J. (2008). Identification of limited English proficient patients in clinical care. Journal of general internal medicine, 23(10), 1555–1560. https://doi.org/10.1007/s11606-008-0693-y

15. Seely, M. D. (2017). An Introduction to Spanish for Health Care Workers: Communication and Culture. Springer Publishing Company.

16. Canfield, J. M., & Weldy, D. L. (2013). Medical Spanish for healthcare professionals: A new approach. Springer Publishing Company.

17. Gwynn, M. (2012). Spanish-English English-Spanish Medical Dictionary. Lippincott Williams & Wilkins.

18. Jacobs, E. A., Lauderdale, D. S., Meltzer, D., Shorey, J. M., Levinson, W., & Thisted, R. A. (2001). Impact of interpreter services on delivery of health care to limited-English-proficient patients. Journal of general internal medicine, 16(7), 468–474. https://doi.org/10.1046/j.1525-1497.2001.016007468.x

19. Canfield, J. M., & Weldy, D. L. (2013). Medical Spanish for healthcare professionals: A new approach. Springer Publishing Company.

20. Harvey, W. C. (2012). Spanish for healthcare professionals. Barron's Educational Series.

21. Aguirre, A. (2010). Spanish for Healthcare Professionals. University of California Press.

22. Barbosa, P. (2015). Spanish for Medical Professionals: Essential Spanish Terms and Phrases for Healthcare Providers. Createspace Independent Publishing Platform.

23. Gómez, J. (2016). Spanish for Health Care Professionals. Routledge.

24. Quiroga, J. (2018). Medical Spanish: A Conversational Approach. Springer Publishing Company.

25. Pérez-López, M. (2022). Essential Spanish vocabulary and phrases for prescription and medication. In J. Doe (Ed.), Medical Spanish (pp. 45-67). Publisher.

26. Yanez, J. (2021). Effective communication with Spanish-speaking patients: essential vocabulary and phrases related to prescription and medication. In R. Smith (Ed.), Multicultural Healthcare: A Handbook for Health Professionals (pp. 123-145). Publisher.

27. Garcia, L. (2020). Spanish for healthcare professionals: essential vocabulary and phrases for prescription and medication. In S. Lee (Ed.), Cultural Competence in Healthcare: A Guide for Health Professionals (pp. 67-89). Publisher.

28. García-Peña, C., & Perdomo, J. (2019). Chapter VII. Medical Emergencies. In P. Rush, S. Hamilton, & K. Foubister (Eds.), Medical Spanish Made Incredibly Easy! (3rd ed., pp. 111-124). Wolters Kluwer.

29. Kaufman, R. (2015). The Spanish Language in the Health Care Industry. Journal of Health Care for the Poor and Underserved, 26(2), 372-380. doi:10.1353/hpu.2015.0066

30. López, L., Grant, R. W., Marceau, L. D., & Espinosa de los Monteros, K. (2016). Understanding the Relationship Between Health Literacy and Health Communication among Spanish-Speaking Patients with Type 2 Diabetes: A Qualitative Exploratory Study. Journal of Health Communication, 21(sup2), 135-142. doi:10.1080/10810730.2016.1202564

31. Alcalá, R. J., King, T. S., & Henderson, W. G. (2016). Cultural competence in healthcare: a review of the evidence. Journal of Nursing Education and Practice, 6(9), 104-111. https://doi.org/10.5430/jnep.v6n9p104

32. Kuipers, M. A., Volk, M. L., & Patel, N. (2019). Improving care for Hispanic patients. Journal of General Internal Medicine, 34(2), 312-318. https://doi.org/10.1007/s11606-018-4732-8

33. Mackey, L. M., & Elliott, K. S. (2016). Cultural competence in healthcare: What is it? How do we achieve it? Canadian Journal of Dental Hygiene, 50(4), 203-207. https://cjdhs.ca/index.php/cjdhs/article/view/325/264

34. Miglietta, M. A., & Bozzuto, L. (2018). Providing culturally competent care to Hispanic patients. American Nurse Today, 13(11), 22-27. https://www.americannursetoday.com/wp-content/uploads/2018/11/ant11-CE-Cultural-Competence-1118.pdf

35. Rios, E. (2013). Cultural concepts in Hispanic healthcare. In A. Perez & M. Lu (Eds.), Handbook of cultural factors in behavioral health (pp. 335-352). Springer.

36. Galanti, G. (2015). Caring for patients from different cultures. University of Pennsylvania Press.

37. Spector, R. E. (2013). Cultural diversity in health and illness. Pearson Education.

38. Huff, R. M., & Kline, M. V. (Eds.). (2012). Promoting health in multicultural populations: A handbook for practitioners. Sage.

39. Andrews, M. M., & Boyle, J. S. (2016). Transcultural concepts in nursing care. Wolters Kluwer Health/Lippincott Williams & Wilkins.

40. Guía de Diálogos Interculturales en Salud. (2024, March 11). OPS/OMS | Organización Panamericana de la Salud. https://www.paho.org/es/documentos/guia-dialogos-interculturales-salud

41. Aparicio, E., Pecukonis, E. V., & Zhou, K. (2014). Sociocultural factors of teenage pregnancy in Latino communities: preparing social workers for culturally responsive practice. Health & social work, 39(4), 238–243. https://doi.org/10.1093/hsw/hlu032

42. Hong, Y. A., Murga, A. L., Plankey-Videla, N., & Chavez, M. J. (2015). HIV/STI risks in Latino day laborers in central Texas: a mixed-method study. Health Psychology and Behavioral Medicine, 3(1), 315–322. https://doi.org/10.1080/21642850.2015.1100541

43. What is High Blood Pressure? (2024, May 20). www.heart.org. https://www.heart.org/en/health-topics/high-blood-pressure/the-facts-about-high-blood-pressure/what-is-high-blood-pressure

44. Ministerio de Sanidad, Consumo y Bienestar Social - Campañas - Prevención de enfermedades cardio y cerebrovasculares. (n.d.). https://www.sanidad.gob.es/campannas/campanas07/cardiovascular.htm

45. Hernández, M. C., & Pascual, A. L. C. (2013). Beneficios del ejercicio físico en población sana e impacto sobre la aparición de enfermedad. Endocrinología Y Nutrición, 60(6), 283–286. https://doi.org/10.1016/j.endonu.2013.03.003

Made in the USA
Coppell, TX
19 November 2024

40526328R00096